THE JOY of YOGA

THE JOY of YOGA

Fifty Sequences for Your Home and Studio Practice

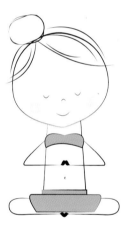

Emma Silverman

Illustrated by

Kerri Frail

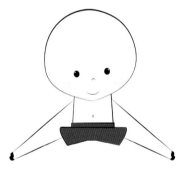

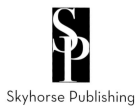

Skyhorse Publishing

Skyhorse Publishing books may be purchased in bulk at special discounts for sales promotion, corporate gifts, fund-raising, or educational purposes. Special editions can also be created to specifications. For details, contact the Special Sales Department, Skyhorse Publishing, 307 West 36th Street, 11th Floor, New York, NY 10018 or info@skyhorsepublishing.com.

Skyhorse® and Skyhorse Publishing® are registered trademarks of Skyhorse Publishing, Inc.®, a Delaware corporation.

www.skyhorsepublishing.com

10 9 8 7 6 5 4 3 2 1

Library of Congress Cataloging-in-Publication Data:

Silverman, Emma.
The joy of yoga: fifty sequences for your home and studio practice / Emma Silverman; illustrated by Kerri Frail.
pages cm
ISBN 978-1-62873-776-9 (hardback)
Ebook ISBN: 978-1-62914-145-9
1. Hatha yoga. 2. Exercise. 3. Health. I. Title.
RA781.7.S546 2014
613.7'046–dc23
2014005912

Cover design by Victoria Bellavia
Cover illustrations by Kerri Frail

Printed in China

Emma:

I dedicate this book to my father, my mother, Danny, Rachel, and Jake—to my family.

Kerri:

To my family, most importantly my sister, for their patience and encouragement throughout this project.

Table of Contents

Introduction

I taught myself yoga out of a book. I was seven years old, a child deprived of television, when I started to poke around my parent's bookcase for entertainment. The book I came across was *The Complete Illustrated Book of Yoga* by Swami Vishnudeananda. It had a pale orange cover with tattered edges and a photo of a serene Indian man meditating, his legs perfectly crossed. Immediately, I was drawn to the pictures inside of the same man rolling his eyes back into his head and sticking his tongue out of his mouth. What I kept coming back to, though, were the many pictures of the different poses or, in Sanskrit, *asanas* shown throughout the pages. The twelve pictures that comprised the Sun Salutations A series changed my life.

That same book, stolen from my parents' shelf (sorry, Mom), is on my own bookshelf today. When I look back at it, I can't imagine how I spent so much time with the book. With the exception of the Sun Salutations images, the book was mostly text and showed incredibly advanced postures. I have some memories of opening to pages at random and trying to do the pose. It's lucky I was young; without any warm-ups, some of those poses I tried at random would probably throw my back out today.

The Joy of Yoga: Fifty Sequences for Your Home and Studio Practice illustrates fifty sequences, warm-ups included, for the newest yogi (of any age) to the yoga teacher. By linking together images of postures in a sequence, an entire yoga class is created. The incredible thing about the practice of yoga is that it can soothe so many physical, mental, and emotional ailments. In these sequences, I tried to address the concerns I regularly hear from my yoga students; there is a sequence for achy hips and also for heartbreak. If you look at the table of contents, I bet you'll find the sequence you need today, in this very moment.

Using this book is simple. Find the sequence that sounds just right, open up to the page, and follow the images. All of the poses have their names listed in Sanskrit and in English. The sequences are complete with warm-ups, complete yoga practices, and cool downs. If you're a little pressed for time (who isn't?), then move through the postures using one breath per pose, unless otherwise noted. If you're looking for a longer practice, you can hold poses for a little longer or combine multiple sequences. Or just take a really long SAVANASA (Relaxation Pose) at the end.

This is a book for the seven-year-old poking around in her (or his) parent's living room and who has never heard of yoga before. This is a book for your grandmother, who has been doing yoga with Jane Fonda since the 1970s, but is looking for something to help her joints. This is a book for the Power Yogi, who throws push-ups inbetween each Sun Salutations. This is a book for you: wherever you are in life or yoga. Welcome to your practice.

Sun Salutations

While the origins of the Sun Salutations (*Surya Namaskar*) might be debatable, the ubiquity of this series in the modern-day yoga studio is definite. The sequence of poses that are shown here are practiced in a style of yoga called *Ashtanga*. That said, numerous variations exist and have similar health and wellness benefits.

There are a couple of reasons that these two sequences are set aside from the rest. Primarily, I will sometimes refer to the Sun Salutations as a step in a larger sequence without writing out each individual pose within the Sun Salutations. That way, you can flip back to this page as a reference while you're still learning the Sun Salutations and later you can move through the flow without needing to check. In addition, this fun and vibrant sequence is usually practiced as a warm-up to other yoga poses, but can be a great stand-alone sequence if you only have a few minutes to spare and could use a yoga wake-up call.

Feel free to add in a Sun Salutations (or twelve) to any sequence in this book. You'll feel more energized, fired up, and radiant—just like the sun!

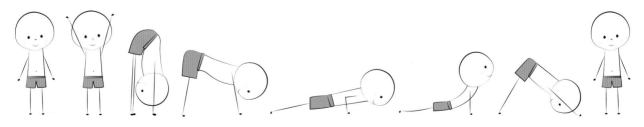

Sun Salutations A

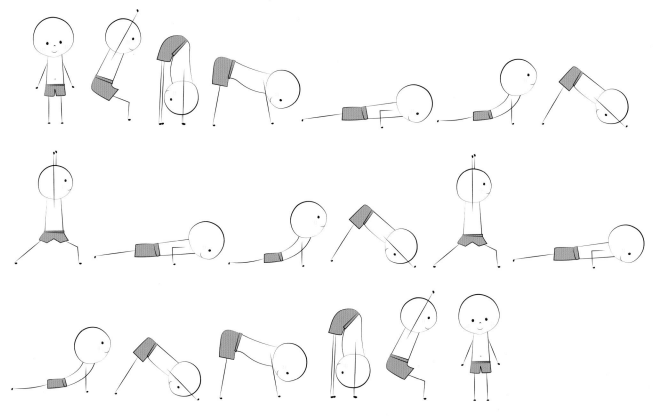

Sun Salutations B

Planes, Trains, and Automobiles

Yoga for Travelers

Airplane Yoga

People ask me all the time about how I became a yoga teacher. The short answer is that I flew in airplanes way too often. I worked as a consultant and had to travel at least four times a month. Pretty quickly, my body assumed the form of an airplane seat. The upside is that I developed a routine to help make flights a little easier on my body. You might look a little weird, but maybe you'll be the only one walking off the plane not aching and hunched over. Then who's the weird-looking one?

1. Breathe deeply into your belly, ribs, and collarbones. Exhale the breath away from your collarbones, rib cage, and belly (Three-Part Yogic Breath). Continue to deeply breathe in and out.

2. In meditative seat: roll the neck, shoulders, wrists, and ankles

3. Interlocking fingers, raise arms above head. Gentle side-to-side motion, side stretch

4. Taking hands to seat head in front of you, let head and neck drop, stretching upper back

5. Move slightly forward in the seat, bringing hands behind you, gentle chest opener

6. Cat/Cow spine in seated position

7. Gentle seated twist using your armrests. Twist both ways.

TURN TO PAGE 6 TO COMPLETE SEQUENCE.

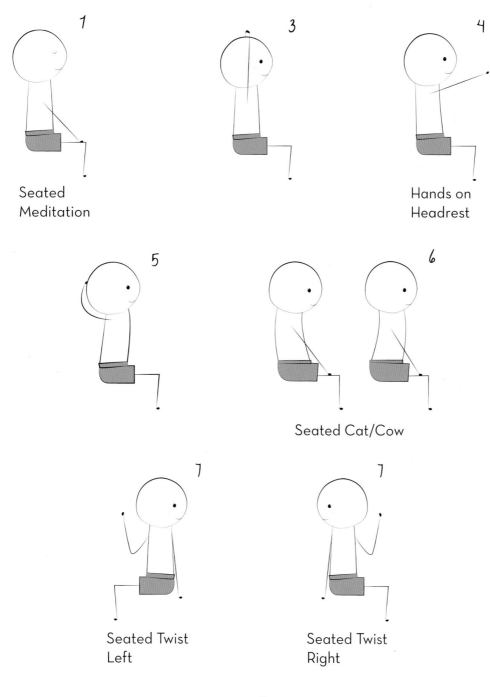

1 Seated Meditation

3

4 Hands on Headrest

5

6 Seated Cat/Cow

7 Seated Twist Left

7 Seated Twist Right

8.   Waiting for the restrooms, *Natarajasana* (Dancer's Pose). Repeat other side.

9.   *Tadasana* (Mountain Pose)

10. *Pavana Muktasana* (Standing Wind Relieving Pose). Repeat other side.

11. *Tadasana*

12. Seated *Tadasana*

13. Repeat all steps whenever the body starts to feel achy

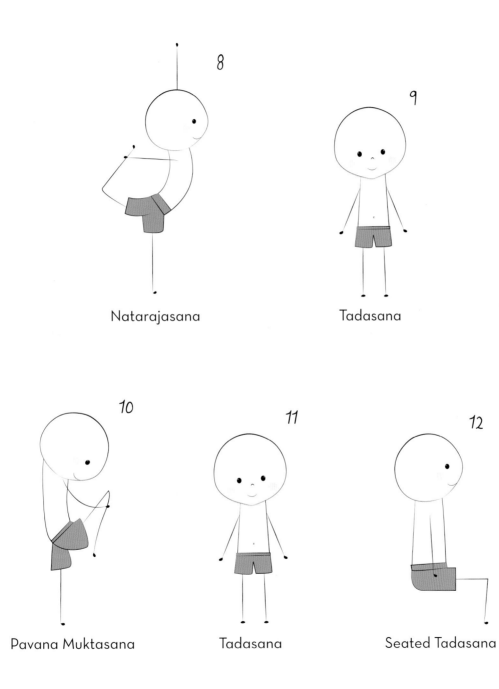

8   Natarajasana

9   Tadasana

10   Pavana Muktasana

11   Tadasana

12   Seated Tadasana

The Road Tripper's Guide to Yoga

Before I moved to Ithaca, New York (my current home), I spent almost a year traveling the United States, visiting cities and searching for a new place to call home. Thirty states later, New York won. In the process, however, I took yoga classes everywhere and had a great time. Whenever there wasn't a studio or classes available, or I just didn't have the time or the money, a regular "home" yoga practice was key to my sanity. Here are some poses for the sore butts, achy lower backs, and the Jack Kerouac in all of us.

1. Meditation
2. *Ardha Matsyendrasana* (Half Seated Twist Pose)
3. Table Top
4. Cat/Cow spine in Table Top
5. *Adho Mukha Svanasana* (Downward Facing Dog Pose), 5 cycles of breath to "pedal" your legs and move
6. Sun Salutations, 6–12 times to get the blood moving
7. *ardha salabhasana* (Half Locust Pose)
8. *salabhasana* (Locust Pose)

Turn to page 10 to complete sequence.

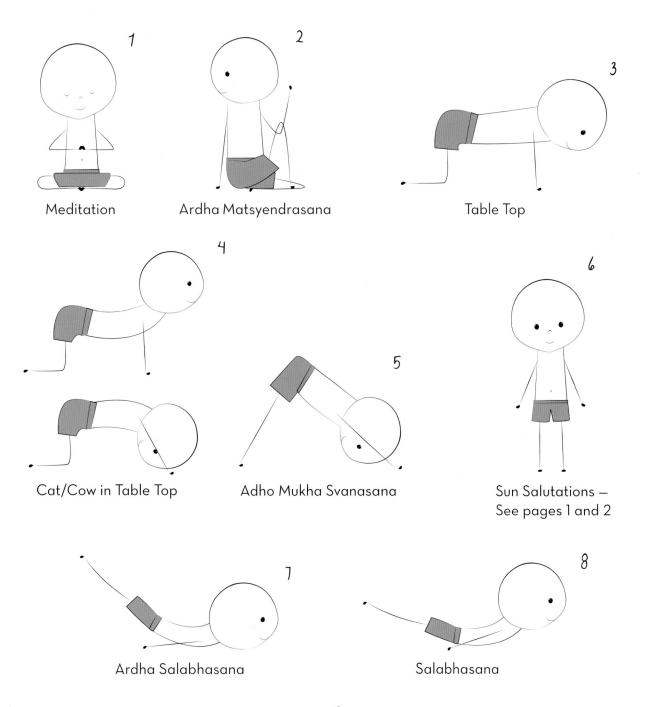

1 Meditation

2 Ardha Matsyendrasana

3 Table Top

4 Cat/Cow in Table Top

5 Adho Mukha Svanasana

6 Sun Salutations –
See pages 1 and 2

7 Ardha Salabhasana

8 Salabhasana

9. *Dhanurasana* (Bow Pose)

10. *Balasana* (Child's Pose)

11. *Adho Mukha Svanasana* (Downward Facing Dog Pose)

12. *Supta kapotasana* (Reclined Pigeon Pose). Repeat other side.

13. *Janu Sirsasana* (Head to Knee Pose)

14. *Parivrtta Janu Sirsasana* (Revolved Head to Knee Pose)

15. *Ardha Matsyendrasana* (Half Seated Twist Pose)

16. Repeat steps 13-15 on other side

17. *Savasana* (Corpse Pose)

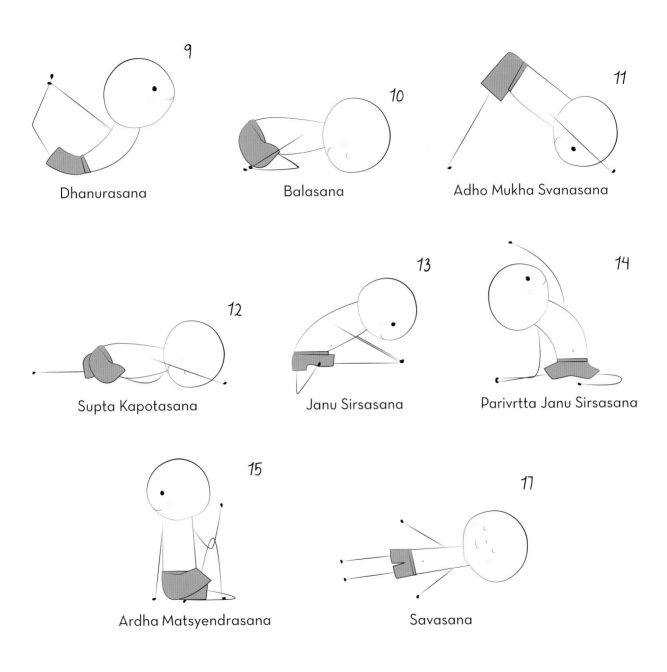

9 Dhanurasana

10 Balasana

11 Adho Mukha Svanasana

12 Supta Kapotasana

13 Janu Sirsasana

14 Parivrtta Janu Sirsasana

15 Ardha Matsyendrasana

17 Savasana

Subway and Train Station Yoga

I used to take yoga classes when I lived in Mexico City. Even discounting the fact that my Spanish was subpar, it was a weird experience. Mexico City is one of the most polluted cities in the world (sorry L.A., you ain't got nothing on this city) and breathing deeply could leave me in a coughing fit. So what does a yoga class look like? Lots and lots of *ujjayi*—or victorious breath—into and out of the nostrils. I would recommend the same for yoga in the subway or on the train platform. Find that deep, sonorous breath into and out of the nose and strike a few poses to let the rest of the commuters know you are not a yogi to mess with.

1. *DEVIASANA* (Goddess Pose or Horse Stance)
2. *Virabhadrasana II* (Warrior II Pose)
3. *DEVIASANA*
4. *Virabhadrasana II*, other side
5. Repeat steps 1-4 coming from side to side for 5-10 rounds of *Ujjayi pranayama* (Victorious Breath)
6. High lunge, bending and straightening front leg
7. *Parsvottanasana* (Intense Side Stretch Pose)
8. Repeat poses 6 and 7 on other side
9. *Prasarita Padottanasana* (Wide-Legged Forward Bend)
10. *Simhasana* (Lion's Pose)

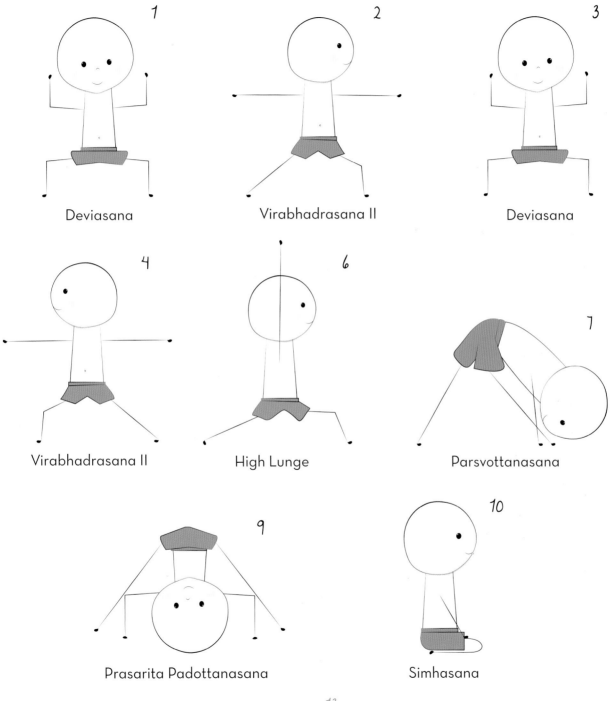

1 Deviasana

2 Virabhadrasana II

3 Deviasana

4 Virabhadrasana II

6 High Lunge

7 Parsvottanasana

9 Prasarita Padottanasana

10 Simhasana

Yoga You Can Do While Waiting for the Bus

The main difference between **Subway and Train Station Yoga** and **Yoga You Can Do While Waiting for the Bus** is how freaky you are allowed to look. While I have seen a man in a Speedo walking around the New York City subway system, I have not seen that same man waiting for the bus (thank goodness). Here are a few gentle stretches that leave you more relaxed and on the right side of crazy.

1. *Tadasana* (Mountain Pose)
2. *Yoga Mudrasana* (Standing Forward Fold with Hands Clasped)
3. *Urdhva Hastasana* (Upward Hands Pose)
4. Breathe between poses 2 and 3, exhaling to step 2, inhaling to step 3
5. *Pavana Muktasana* (Standing Wind Relieving Pose). Repeat on other side.
6. Gentle *Natarajasana* (Dancer's Pose). Repeat on other side.
7. Standing Cat/Cow (hands on knees)
8. *Tadasana*

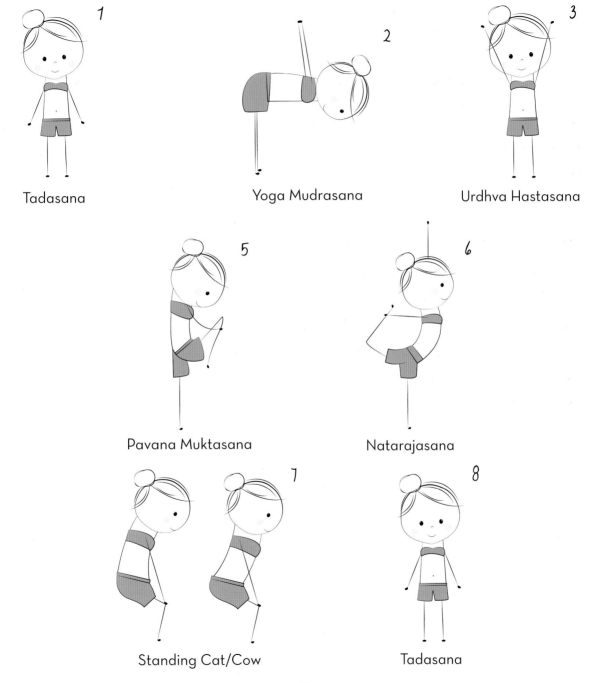

1 Tadasana

2 Yoga Mudrasana

3 Urdhva Hastasana

5 Pavana Muktasana

6 Natarajasana

7 Standing Cat/Cow

8 Tadasana

Immunity-Boosting Yoga Sequence

With all this travel, we wouldn't want to get sick, would we? No, we wouldn't. Let's wrap things up, then, with a sequence that does all the right things to keep you on your toes whether on the road or at home. Really, any yoga practice is an immunity booster. People with more stress in their lives are more susceptible to getting sick; people who have a steady yoga and meditation practice are less likely to have high levels of stress. A full-body workout also moves lymph and helps reoxygenate the blood. That being said, there are poses that focus more on the cold-fighting systems of the body than others. Forward bends, back bends, and twists (compressing the digestive tract) will all do the trick nicely.

1. *SUKHASANA* (Easy Pose)
2. *BALASANA* (Child's Pose). Hold for 1 minute, or 5 cycles of breath.
3. Gentle *BHUJANGASANA* (Cobra Pose)
4. Move between *BHUJANASANA* to *BALASANA*. Repeat 5 times.
5. *GOMUKHASANA* (Cow Face Pose). Repeat on other side.
6. Cat/Cow spine in Table Top
7. *ADHO MUKHA SVANASANA* (Downward Facing Dog Pose). Hold for 1–2 minutes.
8. *URDHVA HASTASANA* (Upward Hands Pose). Hold for 5 cycles of breath.
9. *TADASANA* (Mountain Pose)
10. Sun Salutations, 5–10 times

TURN TO PAGE 18 TO COMPLETE SEQUENCE.

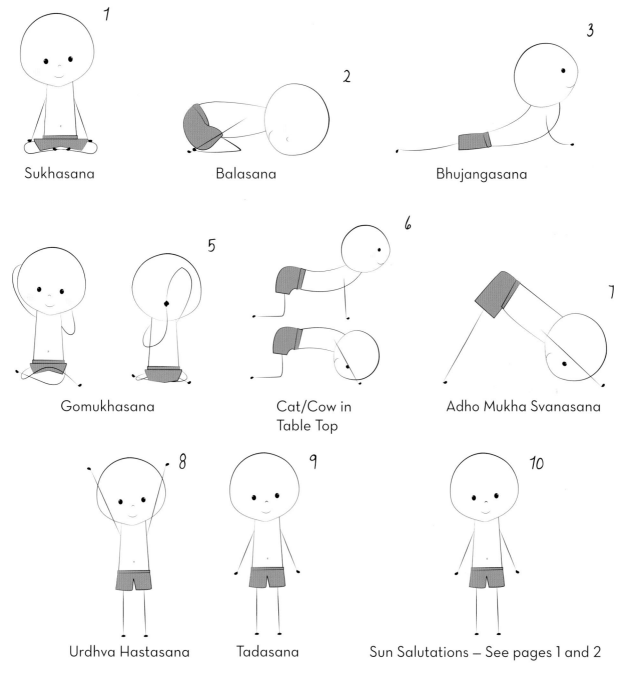

1 Sukhasana

2 Balasana

3 Bhujangasana

Gomukhasana

5

6 Cat/Cow in Table Top

7 Adho Mukha Svanasana

8 Urdhva Hastasana

9 Tadasana

10 Sun Salutations — See pages 1 and 2

17

11. *Uttanasana* (Standing Forward Fold). Hold for 1–2 minutes.

12. *Adho Mukha Svanasana*

13. *Parivrtta Alanasana* (Twisted High Lunge Pose)

14. *Parsvottanasana* (Intense Side Stretch Pose)

15. Repeat steps 12–14 for other leg

16. *Adho Mukha Svanasana*

17. *Savasana* (Corpse Pose)

18. *Supta Pavana Muktasana* (Reclined Wind Relieving Pose)

19. *Supta Matsyendrasana* (Reclined Twist Pose)

20. Repeat steps 18 and 19 on other side

21. *Viparita Karani* (Legs up the Wall Pose)

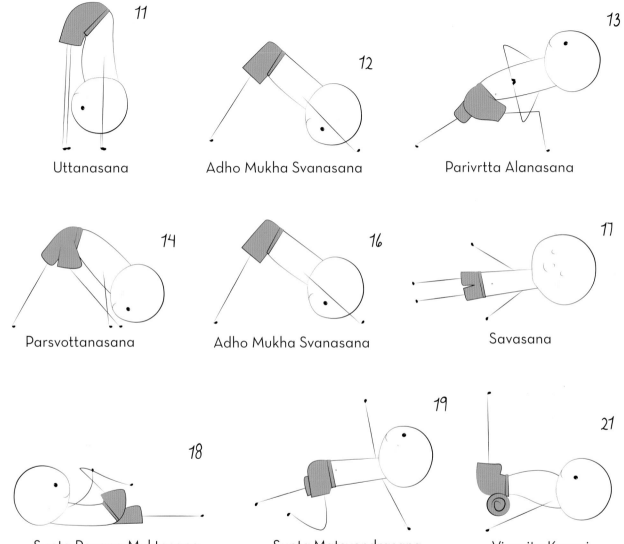

Uttanasana

Adho Mukha Svanasana

Parivrtta Alanasana

Parsvottanasana

Adho Mukha Svanasana

Savasana

Supta Pavana Muktasana

Supta Matsyendrasana

Viparita Karani

Around the House

Yoga to Do at Home

Yoga You Can Do While Waiting for Water to Boil

Of course, when I say "waiting for water to boil," I actually mean, "Waiting for water to boil so you can make homemade Kombucha."

Let's say your Kombucha needs about three and a half quarts of water. That should give us about five minutes to practice yoga. With that kind of time on our hands, better quit reading and get practicing. Here's a routine for when you only have five minutes of time but need five hours worth of energizing!

1. *Tadasana* (Mountain Pose)
2. Inhale to lift your hands to *Urdhva Hastasana* (Upward Hands Pose)
3. Exhale to lower your hands to *Tadasana*
4. Repeat steps 2 and 3 for 1 minute
5. *Virabhadrasana I* (Warrior I Pose)
6. *Virabhadrasana II* (Warrior II Pose)
7. *Deviasana* (Goddess Pose or Horse Stance)
8. *Prasarita Padottanasana* (Wide-Legged Forward Bend)
9. Repeat steps 5 and 6 with other leg
10. *Tadasana*

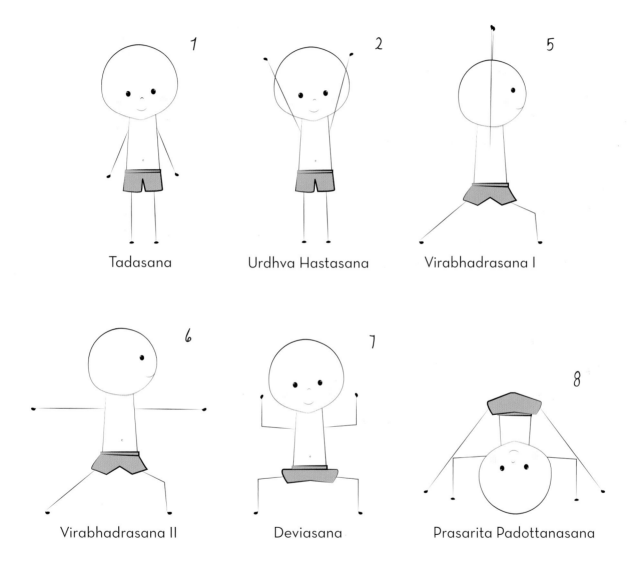

1 Tadasana

2 Urdhva Hastasana

5 Virabhadrasana I

6 Virabhadrasana II

7 Deviasana

8 Prasarita Padottanasana

Yoga up against the Wall

There are lots of great reasons to use a wall during your yoga practice. Maybe you're just starting to find your feet in standing balance poses and you need something to hold onto. Maybe you're looking for something to reinforce your posture. Or maybe you're just looking for a new way to spice up your yoga practice. Whatever the reason, here is a great sequence made even greater by the use of your nearest wall.

1. *Sukhasana* (Easy Pose)
2. *Dandasana* (Staff Pose). Take your back to the wall; notice what parts of your back are touching the wall and which parts are off.
3. *Paschimottanasana* (Seated Forward Fold)
4. *Tadasana* (Mountain Pose)
5. Face the wall. *Uttanasana* (Standing Forward Fold)
6. *Urdhva Hastasana* (Upward Hands Pose)
7. *Ardha Chandrasana* (Balancing Half Moon). Repeat other side.
8. *Virabhadrasana III* (Warrior III Pose) with foot pressing into the wall. Repeat other side.
9. *Dandayamana Janushirasana* (Standing Head to Knee Pose) with foot pressing into the wall. Repeat on other side.
10. *Supta Baddha Konasana* (Reclined Bound Angle Pose), with torso on floor and legs on wall.
11. *Supta Upavistha Konasana* (Reclined Wide Legged Forward Fold) with torso on floor and legs on wall
12. *Viparita Karani* (Legs up the Wall Pose). Hold for 5-10 minutes.

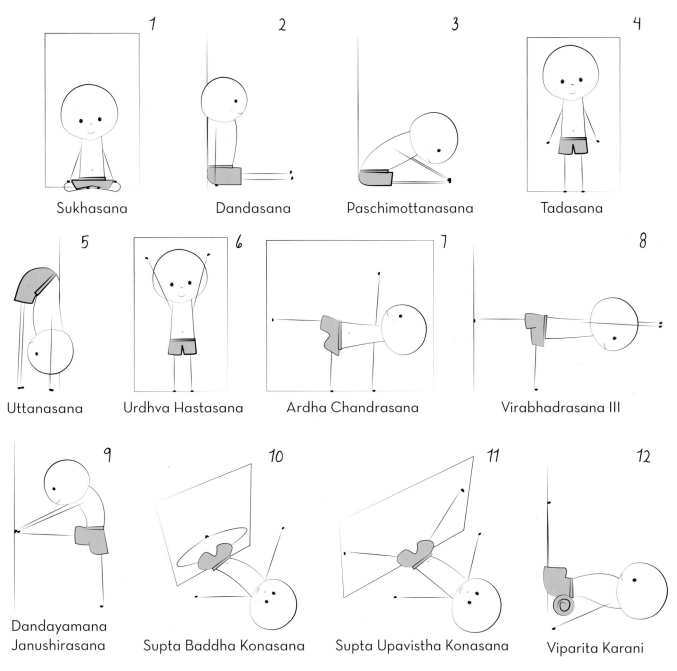

1 Sukhasana

2 Dandasana

3 Paschimottanasana

4 Tadasana

5 Uttanasana

6 Urdhva Hastasana

7 Ardha Chandrasana

8 Virabhadrasana III

9 Dandayamana Janushirasana

10 Supta Baddha Konasana

11 Supta Upavistha Konasana

12 Viparita Karani

Yoga for First Thing in the Morning

I am NOT a morning person. When other people might jump out of bed with a song, I'm more likely to throw a sweatshirt over my eyes and pray I fall back to sleep. Although I usually need to drag myself to my mat, I'm always glad that I did. Even if you aren't a morning person, I dare you to give it a try. A good yoga practice can help regulate the flow of adrenaline in the body and be more effective than your regular 64-oz cup of coffee.

1. *Savasana* (Corpse Pose)
2. *Supta Matsyendrasana* (Reclined Twist Pose). Repeat other side.
3. *Balasana* (Child's Pose). Hold for 2–3 minutes.
4. *Adho Mukha Svanasana* (Downward Facing Dog Pose)
5. *Urdhva Mukha Svanasana* (Upward Facing Dog Pose)
6. Move between steps 4 and 5, warming up the body
7. Facing the direction of the rising sun, enjoy 12 *Surya Namaskar A* (Sun Salutations A).
8. *Balasana*. Hold 2–3 minutes.
9. *Supta Matsyendrasana* (Reclined Twist Pose). Repeat other side.
10. Meditation

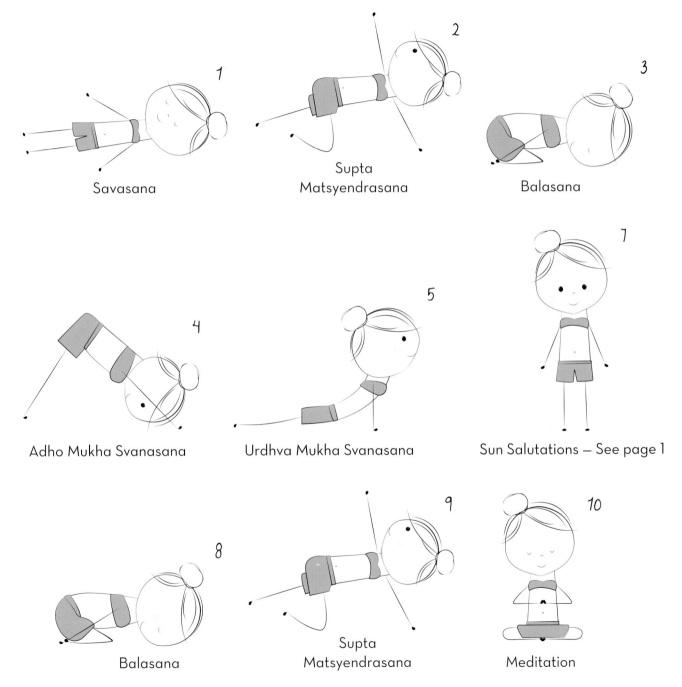

1 Savasana

2 Supta Matsyendrasana

3 Balasana

4 Adho Mukha Svanasana

5 Urdhva Mukha Svanasana

7 Sun Salutations — See page 1

8 Balasana

9 Supta Matsyendrasana

10 Meditation

27

Yoga to Put You to Sleep

If you didn't have time for a complete yoga practice during the day (which helps promote easy and restful sleep at night), try a shorter practice right before you head to bed. This calming practice activates the parasympathetic nervous system (the branch of the autonomic nervous system that mediates the relaxation response), decreases your blood pressure, and slows your heart rate. Before you know it, you'll be counting yogi sheep.

1. *SUKHASANA* (Easy Pose)

2. *NADI SHODANA PRANAYAMA* (Alternate Nostril Breathing), 5 minutes

3. *PASCHIMOTTANASANA* (Seated Forward Fold)

4. *BADDHA KONASANA* (Bound Angle Pose)

5. *SUPTA BADDHA KONASANA* (Reclined Bound Angle Pose). Note: Use lots of pillows if necessary, as with all poses.

6. *JANU SIRSASANA* (Head to Knee Pose). Repeat other side.

7. *SETU BANDHASANA* (Gentle Bridge Pose)

8. *SARVANGASANA* (Shoulderstand Pose)

9. *VIPARITA KARANI* (Legs up the Wall Pose)

10. *SAVASANA* (Corpse Pose) under the covers!

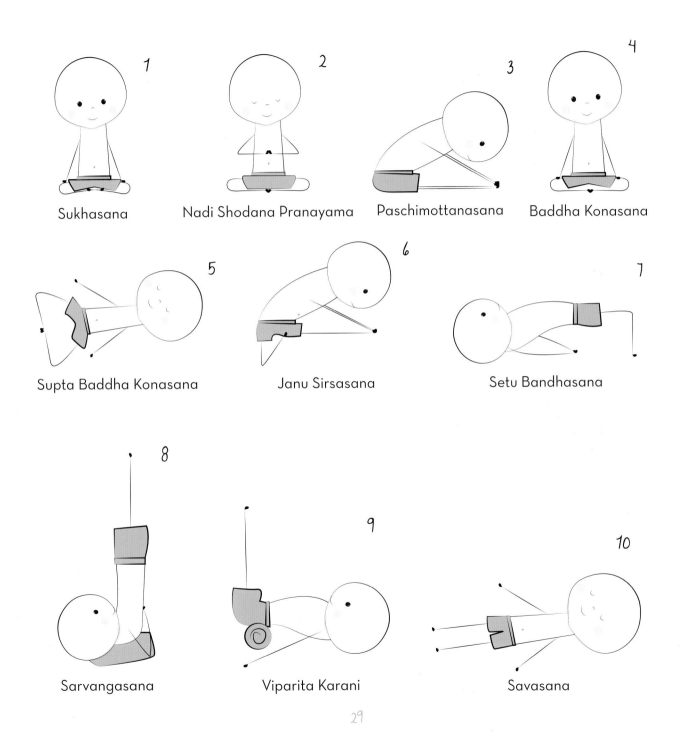

1 Sukhasana

2 Nadi Shodana Pranayama

3 Paschimottanasana

4 Baddha Konasana

5 Supta Baddha Konasana

6 Janu Sirsasana

7 Setu Bandhasana

8 Sarvangasana

9 Viparita Karani

10 Savasana

Yoga after a Long Day

I think there are two kinds of Long Days. One kind of long day has you constantly on your feet, running from place to place, and exhausted from keeping track of every small detail of your big, busy life. The other kind of long day involves so many hours in front of a computer screen that your eyes and brain hurt. Good thing there's a yoga practice that works for YOUR long day, whatever it looked like. I encourage you to practice as much as you can with your eyes closed. It will help create more body awareness and also give your poor eyes a well-deserved break.

1. *Balasana* (Child's Pose). Hold for ten slow cycles of breath.
2. Table Top
3. Extend opposite arm and leg. Repeat other side.
4. *Vyaghrasana* (Tiger Pose). Repeat other side.
5. *Adho Mukha Svanasana* (Downward Facing Dog Pose). "Pedal" your heels, bending one knee and then the other.
6. *Uttanasana* (Standing Forward Fold). Hold for five slow cycles of breath.
7. *Malasana* (Seated Squat)
8. Move between step 6 on exhale and step 7 on inhale, 5-10 times
9. *Sukhasana* (Easy Seated Pose)

Turn to page 32 to complete sequence.

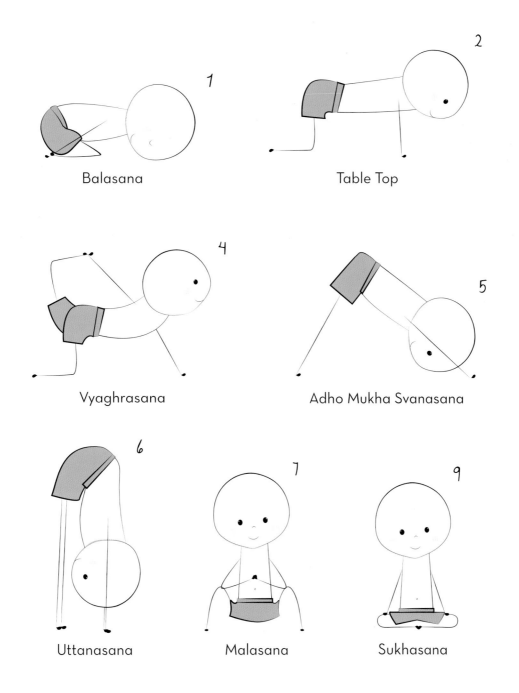

1
Balasana

2
Table Top

4
Vyaghrasana

5
Adho Mukha Svanasana

6
Uttanasana

7
Malasana

9
Sukhasana

10. *Ardha Matsyendrasana* (Half Seated Twist Pose). Repeat other side.

11. *Paschimottanasana* (Seated Forward Fold)

12. *Halasana* (Plow Pose)

13. *Sarvangasana* (Shoulderstand Pose)

14. *Matsyasana* (Fish Pose)

15. *Supta Matsyendrasana* (Reclined Twist Pose). Repeat other side.

16. *Viparita Karani* (Legs up the Wall Pose) for 5-10 minutes

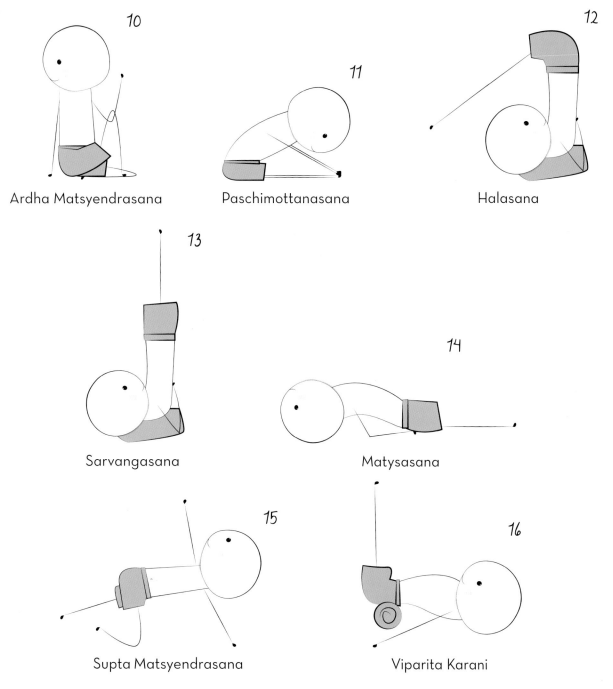

10 Ardha Matsyendrasana

11 Paschimottanasana

12 Halasana

13 Sarvangasana

14 Matysasana

15 Supta Matsyendrasana

16 Viparita Karani

A Restorative Yoga Sequence

Restorative yoga, generally speaking, uses lots of props and is designed to let the body open and relax passively. Hold these poses for 3-5 minutes and focus the breath on the area where you feel the stretch/opening. I prefer restorative practices later in the day; relaxing helps me unwind and prepare for sleeping and settling in for the night. Of course, you can follow this sequence whenever it is you want to relax, renew, and restore.

1. *Sukhasana* (Easy Pose)
2. *Dirgha* and *Ujjayi Pranayama* (Three Part Breath and Victorious Breath). Come back to this breath often throughout this practice.
3. *Baddha Konasana* (Bound Angle Pose). Put pillows or blankets under knees or sitting bones if needed.
4. *Gomukhasana* (Cow Face Pose) with arms resting in a comfortable place
5. *Upavistha Konasana* (Seated Wide Angle Forward Bend)
6. Repeat step 4 with other leg on top
7. *Supta Kapotasana* (Reclined Pigeon Pose). Repeat other side. A pillow under the hip can feel nice here.

Turn to page 36 to complete sequence.

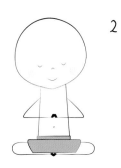
1

Sukhasana

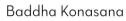
2

Pranayama

3

Baddha Konasana

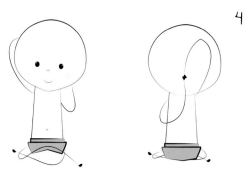
4

Gomukhasana

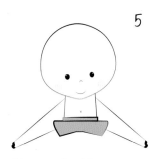
5

Upavistha Konasana

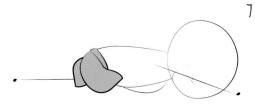
7

Supta Kapotasana

8. Cat/Cow spine in Table Top, 6-10 breaths

9. *Supta Baddha Konasana* (Reclined Bound Angle Pose)

10. *Supta Virasana* (Reclining Heroes Pose)

11. *Supta Matsyendrasana* (Reclined Twist Pose). Repeat on other side.

12. *Viparita Karani* (Legs up the Wall Pose). Hold for 5-10 minutes.

13. *Savasana* (Corpse Pose). Hold for twice your usual length.

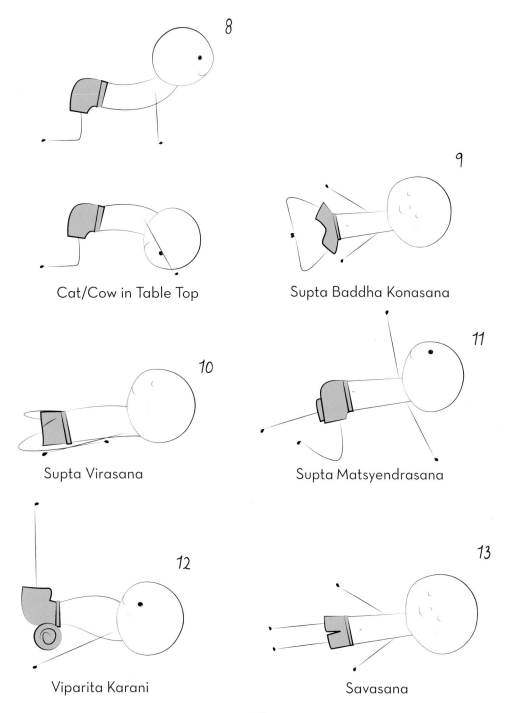

8

9

Cat/Cow in Table Top

Supta Baddha Konasana

10

11

Supta Virasana

Supta Matsyendrasana

12

13

Viparita Karani

Savasana

Punching the Time Clock

Yoga You Can Do At and After Work

Yoga in Your Office Chair

This sequence is for that moment when your eyes start to glaze over, the blood starts to pool in your behind, and your back starts to hurt from hunching over your keyboard. Giving yourself a quick yoga break will clear your mind of clutter and your body of aches. In the end, you'll probably be more productive, and—at the very least—a lot happier.

1. Begin in seated *Tadasana* (Mountain Pose)
2. Bring the arms into *Garundasana* (Eagle Pose). Inhale to lift the arms to the sky, exhale to lower toward the floor. Repeat 5-10 times.
3. Seated twist toward the right
4. Repeat step 3 with other arm underneath.
5. Seated twist toward the left
6. Extend your right leg forward, parallel to the floor, and off of the ground (*Utthita Hasta Padangusthasana*). Note: Use the chair for support, grasping the seat with your hands.
7. Cross your right leg over your left to the best of your mobility.
8. Exhale to fold over the legs.
9. Repeat steps 6-8 on other side.
10. Seated *Garundasana* (Eagle Pose). Repeat other side.
11. Seated *meditation*. Note: Keep eyes closed to help reduce strain.

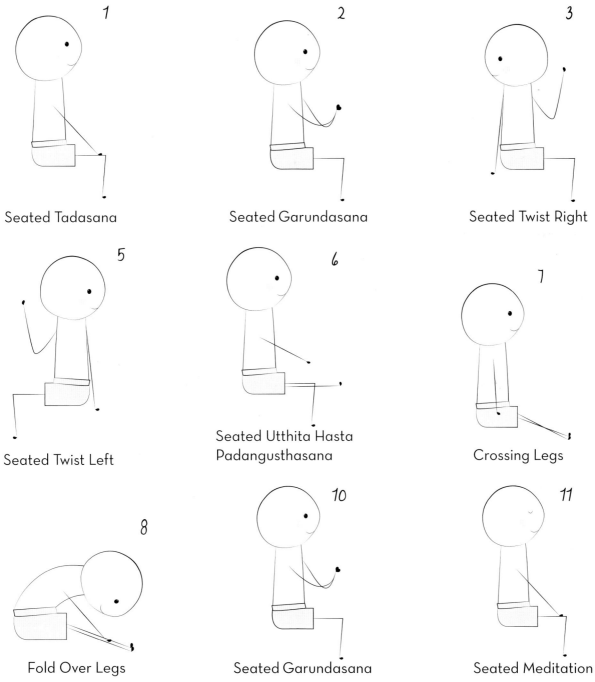

1

Seated Tadasana

2

Seated Garundasana

3

Seated Twist Right

5

Seated Twist Left

6

Seated Utthita Hasta
Padangusthasana

7

Crossing Legs

8

Fold Over Legs

10

Seated Garundasana

11

Seated Meditation

Yoga for Desk Jockeys

Sometimes, after a really long day in front of a computer, all I want to do is become one with my couch and watch THE DAILY SHOW. Really, what I should be doing is a vigorous yoga practice to get myself moving after too much time sitting down and staring at a screen. So while this isn't the sequence to do in your cube, it's perfect for the yogi who spends far too much time in aforementioned cube. If it's nice outside, bring your mat outside to get some fresh air while you practice. If a bug gets on you, well, at least it's not on your hard drive.

1. *TADASANA* (Mountain Pose)

2. *SURYA NAMASKAR A* (Sun Salutations A). Repeat 5 times.

3. *SURYA NAMASKAR B* (Sun Salutations B). Repeat 5 times.

4. *VIRABHADRASANA II* (Warrior II Pose)

5. *BADDHA VIRABHADRASANA* (Humble Warrior Pose)

6. *VIRABHADRASANA II* (Warrior II Pose)

7. *UTTHITA PARSVAKONASANA* (Extended Side Angle)

8. *VIRABHADRASANA II* (Warrior II Pose)

9. *VIPARITA VIRABHADRASANA* (Peaceful Warrior Pose)

TURN TO PAGE 44 TO COMPLETE SEQUENCE.

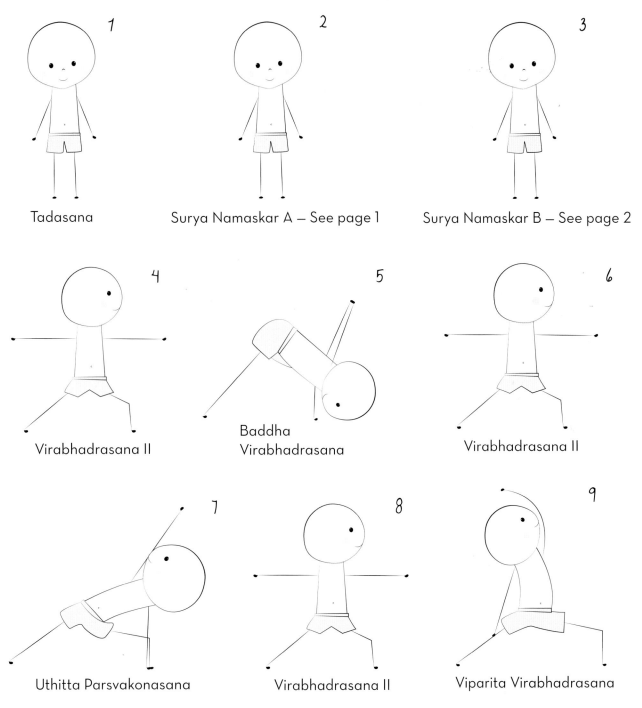

1 Tadasana

2 Surya Namaskar A — See page 1

3 Surya Namaskar B — See page 2

4 Virabhadrasana II

5 Baddha Virabhadrasana

6 Virabhadrasana II

7 Uthitta Parsvakonasana

8 Virabhadrasana II

9 Viparita Virabhadrasana

10. *SURYA NAMASKAR* A

11. Repeat steps 4–10 on other side

12. *TADASANA*

13. *PRASARITA PADOTTANASANA* (Wide-Legged Forward Bend)

14. *SUKHASANA* (Easy Seat)

15. *PASCHIMOTTANASANA* (Seated Forward Fold)

16. *PURVOTTANASANA* (Reverse Plank Pose)

17. *BALASANA* (Child's Pose)

18. *SUPTA MATSYENDRASANA* (Reclined Twist Pose). Repeat other side.

19. *SAVASANA* (Corpse Pose)

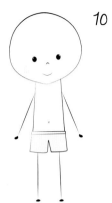

10

Surya Namaskar A — See page 1

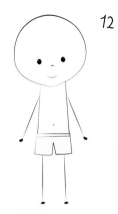

12

Tadasana

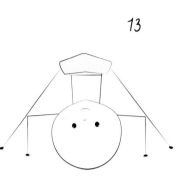

13

Prasarita Padottanasana

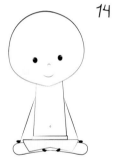

14

Sukhasana

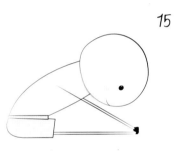

15

Paschimottanasana

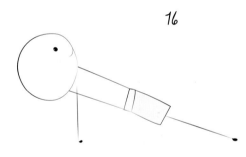

16

Purvottanasana

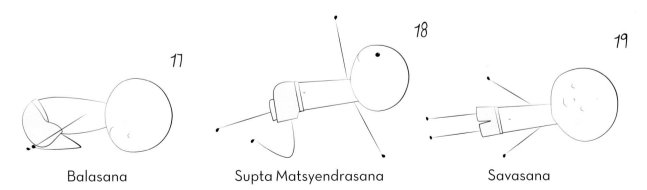

17

Balasana

18

Supta Matsyendrasana

19

Savasana

Yoga for Busy People

I remember when, back in the old days, I used to ask people how they were and they answered, "Good." Now, whenever I ask people how they are doing, they always seem to answer, "Busy, but good." When the world seems like it's spinning too quickly, step back for a moment. Ask yourself: which of these things that are keeping me so busy are really important? Which are my energetic black holes? No matter how much energy I put in, I get nothing back. Take a few minutes of self-reflection in this quick yoga practice, because even busy people need their yoga fix.

1. *SAVASANA* (Corpse Pose)
2. *SUPTA MATSYENDRASANA* (Reclined Twist Pose)
3. *SETU BANDHASANA* (Bridge Pose). Hold for 1-2 minutes.
4. *BALASANA* (Child's Pose)
5. *PARIGHASANA* (Gate Pose)
6. Cat/Cow spine in Table Top

TURN TO PAGE 48 TO COMPLETE SEQUENCE.

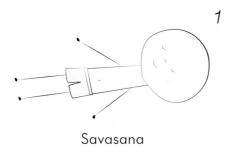

1

Savasana

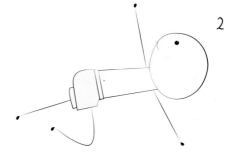

2

Supta Matsyendrasana

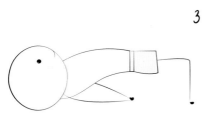

3

Setu Bandhasana

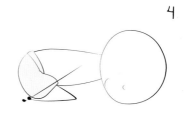

4

Balasana

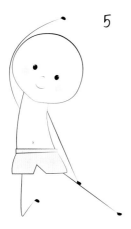

5

Parighasana

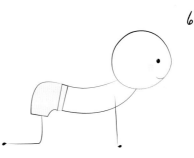

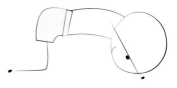

6

Cat/Cow in Table Top

47

7. Repeat *PARIGHASANA* on other side

8. *USTRASANA* (Camel Pose)

9. *VAJRASANA* (Diamond Pose)

10. *USTRASANA* (Camel Pose)

11. *PASCHIMOTTANASANA* (Seated Forward Fold)

12. *PURVOTTANASANA* (Reverse Plank Pose)

13. *SAVASANA* (Corpse Pose)

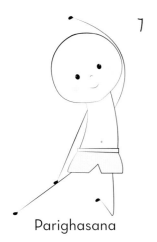

7

Parighasana

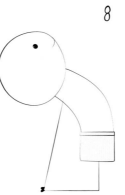

8

Ustrasana

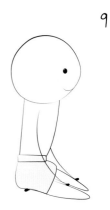

9

Vajrasana

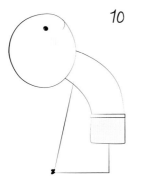

10

Ustrasana

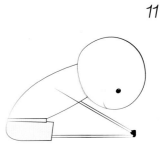

11

Paschimottanasana

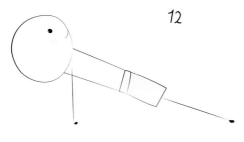

12

Purvottanasana

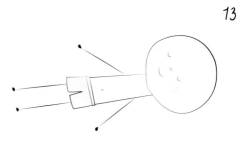

13

Savasana

Yoga for People Who Type Too Much

For the first couple thousand or so years of existence, human beings didn't sit in front of computers and type all day. Accordingly, our bodies are still adjusting to the pressures of sitting, staring at screens. and moving our fingers in the same repeated patterns all day almost every day of the week. This is a sequence to help you out while evolution catches up with us. It releases eye strain, de-tweaks the back, and stretches out the arms and wrists.

1. *Tadasana* (Mountain Pose)
2. *Yoga Mudrasana* (Standing Forward Fold with Hands Interlaced Behind Back)
3. *Urdhva Hastasana* (Upward Hands Pose)
4. *Parsvottanasana* (Intense Side Stretch Pose). Repeat other side.
5. *Garundasana* (Eagle Pose). Repeat other side.
6. *Trikonasana* (Triangle Pose). Repeat other side.
7. *Prasarita Padottanasana* (Wide-Legged Forward Bend). Note: Add Yoga Mudra hands (interlaced) for extra wrist release.
8. *Malasana* (Seated Squat)
9. *Baddha Konasana* (Bound Angle Pose)
10. *Gomukhasana* (Cow Face Pose). Repeat other side.
11. *Ardha Matsyendrasana* (Half Seated Twist Pose). Repeat other side.
12. *Sukhasana* (Seated Meditation) with eyes closed

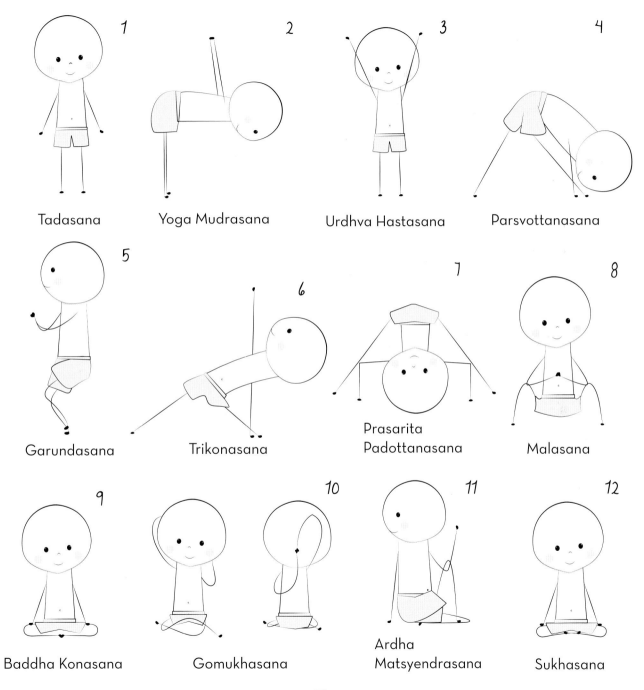

1 Tadasana

2 Yoga Mudrasana

3 Urdhva Hastasana

4 Parsvottanasana

5 Garundasana

6 Trikonasana

7 Prasarita Padottanasana

8 Malasana

9 Baddha Konasana

10 Gomukhasana

11 Ardha Matsyendrasana

12 Sukhasana

51

Midday Pick-Me-Up

Instead of your twelfth trip to the lounge for some stale coffee, why not try a quick yoga routine to wake up your brain and body? This sequence can be done on the sly in the office to help stimulate your adrenal glands (which regulate the flow of adrenaline in the body) and provide you with more clarity than that espresso you were reaching for.

1. *Uttanasana* (Standing Forward Fold). Hold for 2-3 minutes.
2. *Urdhva Hastasana* (Upward Hands Pose). Note: Reach one hand higher and then the other, alternating side stretches.
3. *Yoga Mudrasana* (Standing Forward Fold with Hands Interlaced Behind Back)
4. Standing Cat/Cow
5. *Utkatasana* (Chair Pose)
6. *Parivrtta Utkatasana* (Revolved Chair Pose). Repeat other side.
7. *Uttanasana* (Standing Forward Fold)

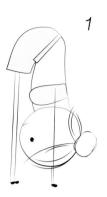

1

Uttanasana

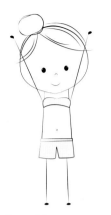

2

Urdhva Hastasana

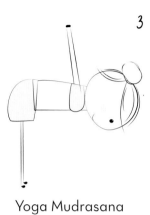

3

Yoga Mudrasana

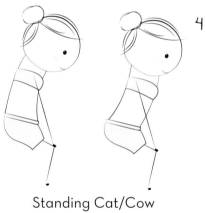

4

Standing Cat/Cow

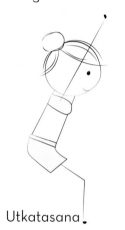

5

Utkatasana

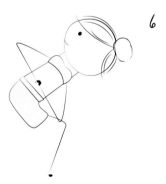

6

Parivrtta Utkatasana

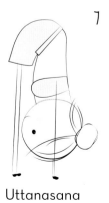

7

Uttanasana

Yoga for Tired Feet

Throughout all of high school and college, I worked as a waitress. I know about tired feet. I know about ankles that swell out of your worn-out Dansko's and threaten to explode. I know about declaring "I'm going to lie down for a while," with no real intention of ever getting up. If you have to run around at work or have just been on your feet all day long, this sequence will give you more energy and stretch out any body aches.

1. *Balasana* (Child's Pose)
2. *Anahatasana* (Extended Puppy Dog Pose)
3. *Adho Mukha Svanasana* (Downward Facing Dog Pose). Take time to pedal your heels and bend the knees.
4. *Bhujangasana* (Cobra Pose)
5. *Salabhasana* (Locust Pose)
6. *Balasana* (Child's Pose)
7. *Adho Mukha Svanasana*

Turn to page 56 to complete sequence.

54

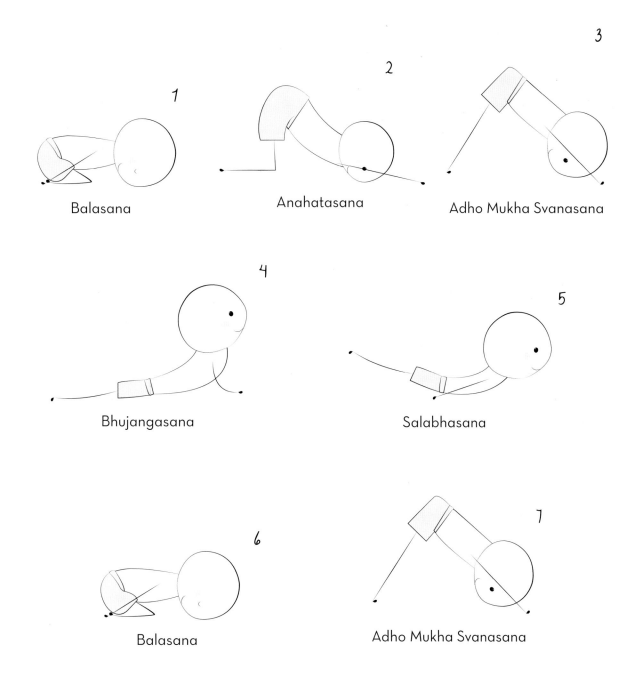

1

Balasana

2

Anahatasana

3

Adho Mukha Svanasana

4

Bhujangasana

5

Salabhasana

6

Balasana

7

Adho Mukha Svanasana

8. *Parsvottanasana* (Intense Side Stretch Pose)

9. *Prasarita Padottanasana* (Wide-Legged Forward Bend)

10. Repeat step 8 with the other leg

11. *Malasana* (Seated Squat Pose)

12. *Janu Sirsasana* (Head to Knee Pose)

13. *Parivrtta Janu Sirsasana* (Revolved Head to Knee Pose)

14. *Upavishta Konasana* (Seated Wide Angle Forward Bend)

15. Repeat steps 12 and 13 with the other leg

16. *Viparita Karani* (Legs up the Wall Pose) for 10-15 minutes

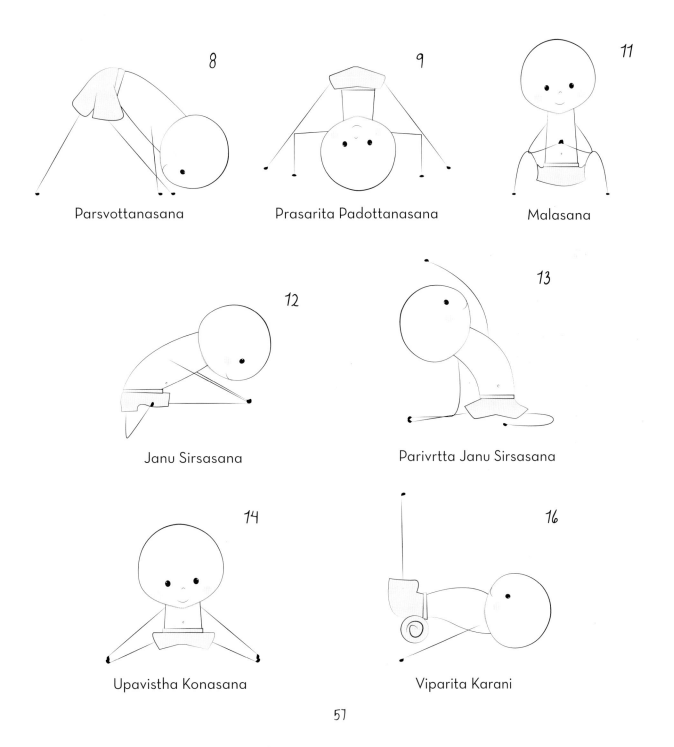

8

Parsvottanasana

9

Prasarita Padottanasana

11

Malasana

12

Janu Sirsasana

13

Parivrtta Janu Sirsasana

14

Upavistha Konasana

16

Viparita Karani

Goddess Yoga

Yoga for the Ladies

Yoga for Menstruation

One of the most common yoga questions I get is: "Can I do yoga if I'm getting my period?" Specifically, ladies often want to know if doing inversions, or going upside down, will somehow affect their cycles (medically proven: it won't). It seems like I'm dodging the question, but the honest answer is to listen to your body. While some yogic traditions (for example, in the Ashtanga style of yoga) advocate for taking breaks while menstruating, I've always maintained my practice and found that it reduces cramping and increases my energy levels. Here is a practice for when your body tells you to move, designed specifically to help with some of the unpleasant side effects that come with a visit from Aunt Flo.

1. *Nadi Shodana Pranayama* (Alternate Nostril Breathing) 5–10 minutes
2. *Upavistha Konasana* (Seated Wide Angle Pose)
3. Cat/Cow spine in Table Top
4. *Bhujangasana* (Cobra Pose)
5. *Adho Mukha Svanasana* (Downward Facing Dog Pose)
6. *Malasana* (Seated Squat Pose)
7. *Supta Pavana Muktasana* (Reclined Wind Relieving Pose). Repeat other side.
8. *Supta Matsyendrasana* (Reclined Twist Pose). Repeat other side.
9. *Supta Baddha Konasana* (Reclined Bound Angle Pose). Hold for a good, long while.
10. *Apanasana* (Knees to Chest on Back)
11. *Viparita Karani* (Legs up the Wall Pose)

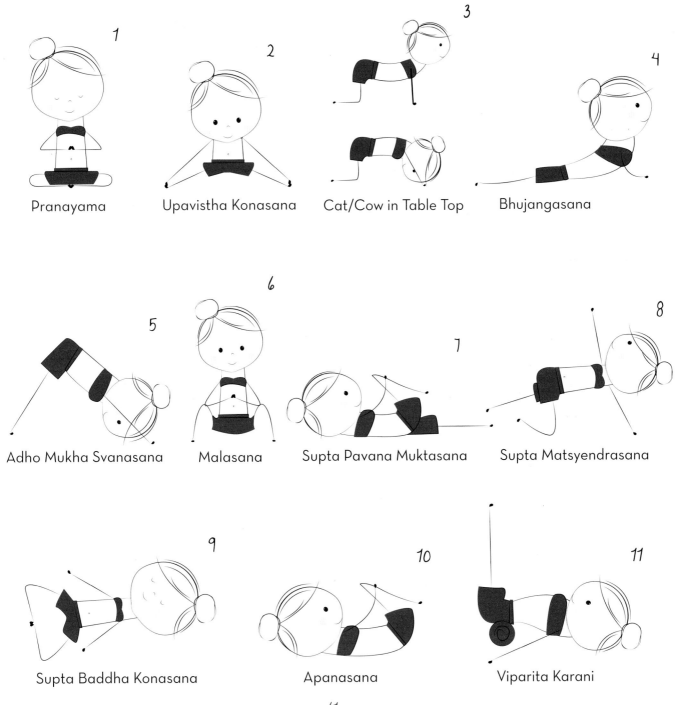

1 Pranayama

2 Upavistha Konasana

3 Cat/Cow in Table Top

4 Bhujangasana

5 Adho Mukha Svanasana

6 Malasana

7 Supta Pavana Muktasana

8 Supta Matsyendrasana

9 Supta Baddha Konasana

10 Apanasana

11 Viparita Karani

Yoga for Pregnancy

Before beginning a home yoga practice while pregnant, I would recommend checking in with your physician and a qualified yoga instructor. The poses recommended for what comes up during different stages of pregnancy change, as will your practice. The sequence I wrote here is appropriate for healthy women at any stage of pregnancy. It can be interesting to practice this sequence once a week, every week and watch how your body changes and adjusts in relation to the postures over time.

1. *SUKHASANA* (Easy Seat)
2. *PARIVRTTA JANU SIRSASANA* (Revolved Head to Knee Pose). Repeat other side.
3. *UPAVISHTA KONASANA* (Seated Wide Angle Forward Bend)
4. *BALASANA* (Child's Pose)
5. Cat/flat spine in Table Top
6. *ANAHATASANA* (Extended Puppy Dog Pose)
7. *TADASANA* (Mountain Pose)
8. *VRKSASANA* (Tree Pose). Repeat other side.
9. *MALASANA* (Seated Squat Pose)
10. *SUPTA BADDHA KONASANA* (Reclined Bound Angle Pose)
11. *VIPARITA KARANI* (Legs up the Wall Pose)

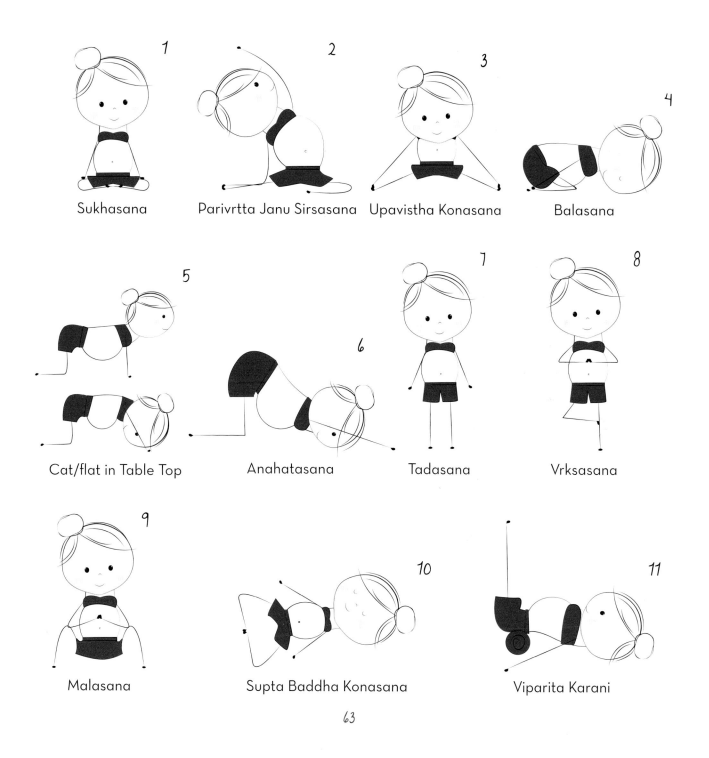

1 Sukhasana

2 Parivrtta Janu Sirsasana

3 Upavistha Konasana

4 Balasana

5 Cat/flat in Table Top

6 Anahatasana

7 Tadasana

8 Vrksasana

9 Malasana

10 Supta Baddha Konasana

11 Viparita Karani

63

Yoga for PMS

I can always tell that I'm about to menstruate when I look down and the Ben & Jerry's is empty and I don't even remember buying the pint. And why does my lower back hurt so much? While I'm at it, what happened to that blissful yogic equanimity? Good thing yoga can help stave off those sugar and salt cravings (and sweat off that pint of ice cream), regulate mood swings, and bring back a little bit of that inner peace.

1. *Balasana* (Child's Pose)
2. *Bhujangasana* (Cobra Pose)
3. *Dhanurasana* (Bow Pose)
4. *Paschimottanasana* (Seated Forward Fold)
5. *Ardha Matsyendrasana* (Half Seated Twist Pose). Repeat other side.
6. *Upavishta Konasana* (Seated Wide Angle Forward Bend)
7. *Apanasana* (Knees to Chest on Back)
8. *Halasana* (Plow Pose)
9. *Sarvangasana* (Shoulderstand Pose)
10. *Apanasana*
11. *Supta Baddha Konasana* (Reclined Bound Angle Pose)

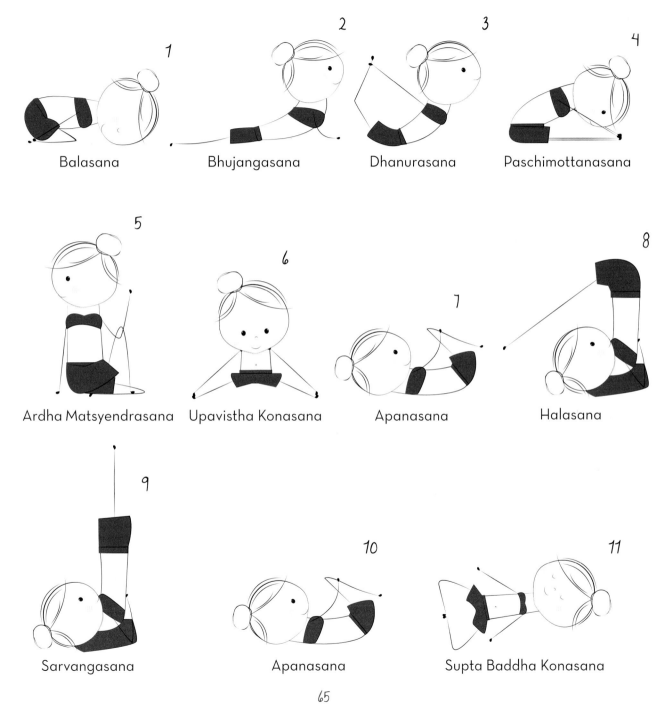

1 Balasana

2 Bhujangasana

3 Dhanurasana

4 Paschimottanasana

5 Ardha Matsyendrasana

6 Upavistha Konasana

7 Apanasana

8 Halasana

9 Sarvangasana

10 Apanasana

11 Supta Baddha Konasana

Yoga for Menopause

I did my Yoga Teacher Training at the Kripalu Institute for Yoga and Health during a particularly cold March. There were a handful of us in our twenties and thirties, but the great majority of the teacher trainees were women in their fifties and sixties. I didn't notice this age gap until I realized the windows were regularly left wide open. "It's so hot in here!" my fellow yogis would say. It wasn't. Also, there was snow on the ground. In the end, I learned to dress warmly for class. This sequence is dedicated to all of my lovely and talented fellow teachers who are, by now, on the other end of menopause. I just wish I could have written it for them then!

1. *SUPTA BADDHA KONASANA* (Reclined Bound Angle Pose)
2. *ANANDA BALASANA* (Happy Baby Pose)
3. *SUPTA MATSYENDRASANA* (Reclined Twist Pose). Note: Take this very gently, as sometimes twists can be warming. Exhale through the mouth as needed.
4. *BALASANA* (Child's Pose)
5. *PASCHIMOTTANASANA* (Seated Forward Fold)
6. *UTTANASANA* (Standing Forward Fold)
7. *MALASANA* (Seated Squat Pose)
8. *VIPARITA KARANI* (Legs up the Wall Pose). Hold for 10-15 minutes.

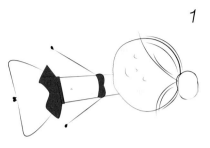

1

Supta Baddha Konasana

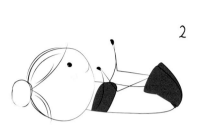

2

Ananda Balasana

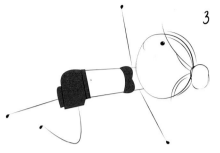

3

Supta Matsyendrasana

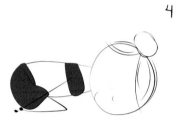

4

Balasana

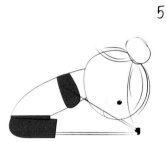

5

Paschimottanasana

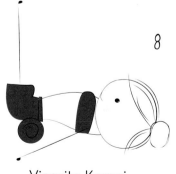

6

Uttanasana

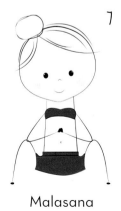

7

Malasana

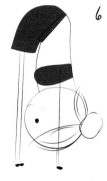

8

Viparita Karani

67

Yoga for Bone Strength

Although bone degeneration becomes more common during menopause (because of reduced estrogen levels), it is always good for us ladies to be aware of strengthening our bones. If you already have been diagnosed with osteoporosis or osteopenia (a precursor to osteoporosis), be very careful with forward folds and twists. If you have any bone fractures, they can be exacerbated by certain yoga positions, so check in with your doctor and yoga instructor before practicing. In general, good osteoporosis-prevention practices put weight on the bones. As you go through this sequence, move slowly and with extra attention to musculoskeletal alignment.

1. *Tadasana* (Mountain Pose)

2. *Vrksasana* (Tree Pose). Repeat on other side.

3. *Pavana Muktasana* (Standing Wind Relieving Pose). Repeat on other side.

4. *Garundasana* (Eagle Pose). Repeat on other side,

5. *Urdhva Hastasana* (Upward Hands Pose)

6. *Utkatasana* (Chair Pose)

7. *Adho Mukha Svanasana* (Downward Facing Dog Pose)

8. *Urdhva Mukha Svanasana* (Upward Facing Dog Pose)

Turn to page 70 to complete sequence.

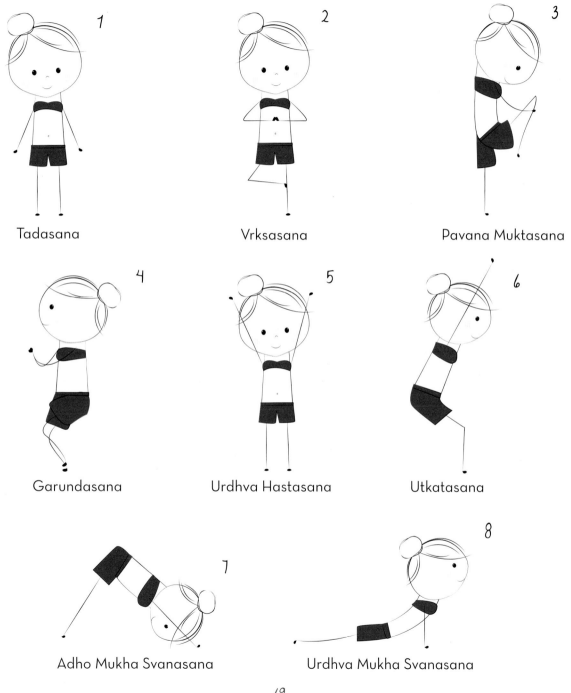

1 Tadasana

2 Vrksasana

3 Pavana Muktasana

4 Garundasana

5 Urdhva Hastasana

6 Utkatasana

7 Adho Mukha Svanasana

8 Urdhva Mukha Svanasana

69

9. *BALASANA* (Child's Pose)

10. *ADHO MUKHA SVANASANA*

11. *VIRABHADRASANA I* (Warrior I Pose)

12. *TRIKONASANA* (Triangle Pose)

13. *UTTHITA PARSVAKONASANA* (Extended Side Angle Pose)

14. *UTTHAN PRISTHASANA* (Lizard Pose)

15. Plank Pose

16. Repeat steps 7-15 on other side of the body

17. *DANDASANA* (Staff Pose)

18. *VIPARITA KARANI* (Legs up the Wall Pose)

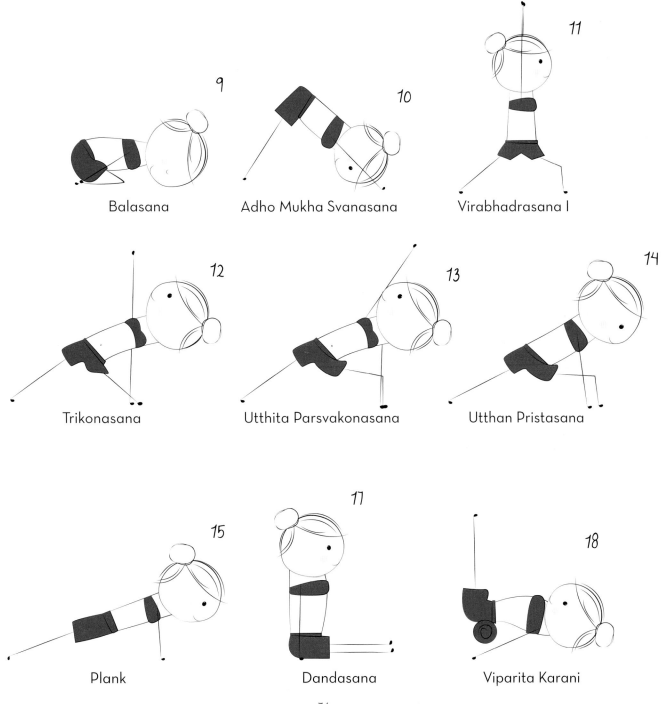

9
Balasana

10
Adho Mukha Svanasana

11
Virabhadrasana I

12
Trikonasana

13
Utthita Parsvakonasana

14
Utthan Pristasana

15
Plank

17
Dandasana

18
Viparita Karani

Just for Fun

Yoga for Everything in Between

A Very Twisty Yoga Sequence

Twists are like the kale of yoga. Just like kale is packed with a ton of health benefits, there are so many ways twists are good for you, it's hard to list them all. Depending on the twist, you might find benefits for managing diabetes, reducing high blood pressure, encouraging fertility, and aiding in digestion. You don't have to put your body into a crazy contortion to enjoy the perks of twisting. Let's get twisted!

1. *Supta Baddha Konasana* (Reclined Bound Angle Pose). Remain here for 1–3 minutes.

2. *Supta Matsyendrasana* (Reclined Twist Pose). Repeat on other side.

3. *Supta Pavana Muktasana* (Reclined Wind Relieving Pose). Repeat on other side.

4. *Apanasana* (Knees to Chest on Back)

5. *Jathara Parivartanasana* (Revolved Belly Pose). Repeat 12 times side to side.

6. *Bhujangasana* (Cobra Pose). Hold for 5 cycles of breath.

7. *Balasana* (Child's Pose)

Turn to page 76 to complete sequence.

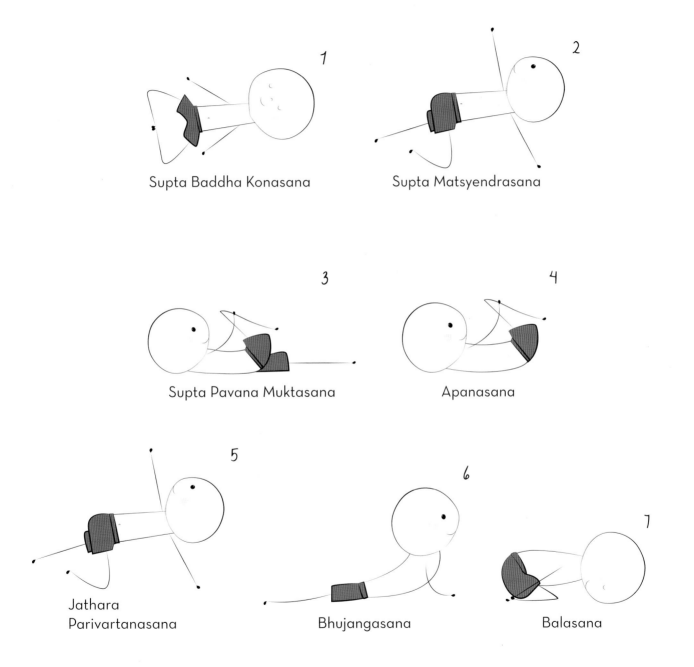

1
Supta Baddha Konasana

2
Supta Matsyendrasana

3
Supta Pavana Muktasana

4
Apanasana

5
Jathara
Parivartanasana

6
Bhujangasana

7
Balasana

8. *Janu Sirsasana* (Head to Knee Pose)

9. *Parivrtta Janu Sirsasana* (Revolved Head to Knee Pose)

10. *Ardha Matsyendrasana* (Half Seated Twist Pose)

11. Repeat steps 8-10 on other side

12. *Baddha Konasana* (Bound Angle Pose)

13. *Gomukhasana* (Cow Face Pose). Repeat on other side.

14. *Savasana* (Corpse Pose)

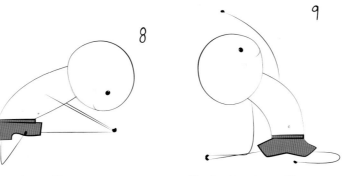

Janu Sirsasana

Parivrtta Janu Sirsasana

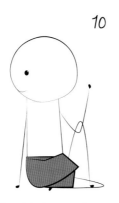

Ardha Matsyendrasana

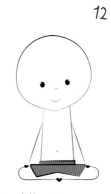

Baddha Konasana

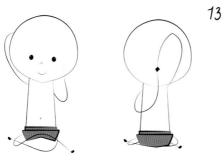

Gomukhasana

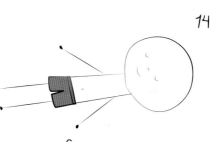

Savasana

77

Yoga Poses that Are Awkward to Do Naked

There was a *SEINFELD* episode a million years ago on the particular subject of how there are just some things best done clothed. Like opening a pickle jar—best done with clothes on. I'm throwing yoga in with opening a pickle jar. These poses are awkward for many reasons: unattractively moving bits, stuff in your face that wasn't meant to be there, and poses that would be terrible if, by accident, a friend or acquaintance walked in. If you want an evening of strange, uncomfortable hilarity, try it out. Just remember to keep the shades drawn.

1. Jump backs. In general.
2. *PADMASANA* (Full Lotus Pose)
3. *JANU SIRSASANA* (Head to Knee Pose)
4. *HANUMANASANA* (Seated Splits)
5. *ADHO MUKHA SVANASANA* (Downward Facing Dog Pose)
6. *DHANURASANA* (Bow) (Especially for men)
7. *SARVANGASANA* (Shoulderstand Pose) (Especially for women)
8. *HALASANA* (Plow Pose) (Especially for women, and very flexible men)
9. *KARNAPIDASANA* (Ear Pressure Pose)
10. *SETU BANDHASANA* (Bridge Pose)
11. *BADDHA KONASANA* (Bound Angle) with forward fold

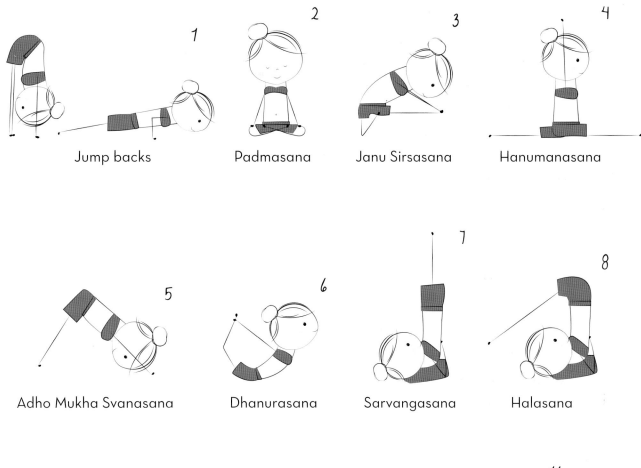

1 Jump backs

2 Padmasana

3 Janu Sirsasana

4 Hanumanasana

5 Adho Mukha Svanasana

6 Dhanurasana

7 Sarvangasana

8 Halasana

9 Karnapidasana

10 Setu Bandhasana

11 Baddha Konasana

Yoga to Love Your Beautiful Self

Some days, from the moment I wake up I avoid the mirror. There's usually no good reason besides feeling GROSS. I'll brush my teeth with my eyes closed if I have to. Then I start to practice yoga and all that goes away. Doesn't matter the pose, doesn't matter the time of day, and definitely doesn't matter if I'm wearing Lululemon. There are, however, poses that are thought to have direct access to brightening our self-image. Lots of powerful, I-am-yogi-hear-me-roar poses will do the trick any day. Love Your Beautiful Self!

1. *TADASANA* (Mountain Pose)

2. *VIRABHADRASANA I* (Warrior I Pose)

3. *VIRABHADRASANA II* (Warrior II Pose)

4. *DEVIASANA* (Horse Stance or Goddess Pose)

5. *KAPALABHATI PRANAYAMA* (Breath of Fire). Note: Continue this breathing technique in *DEVIASANA* for 1 minute.

6. *PRASARITA PADOTTANASANA* (Wide-Legged Forward Bend)

7. Repeat steps 2–6 on other side

8. *TADASANA*

9. *ADHO MUKHA SVANASANA* (Downward Facing Dog Pose)

10. *ALANASANA* (High Lunge Pose) with right foot forward

TURN TO PAGE 82 TO COMPLETE SEQUENCE.

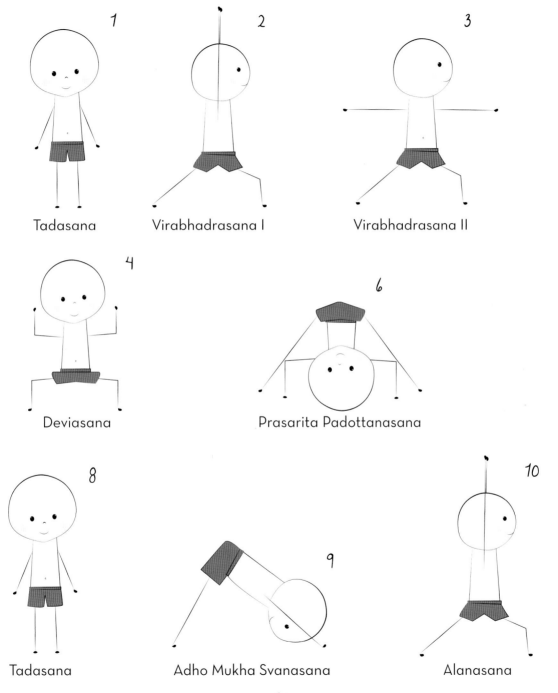

1 Tadasana

2 Virabhadrasana I

3 Virabhadrasana II

4 Deviasana

6 Prasarita Padottanasana

8 Tadasana

9 Adho Mukha Svanasana

10 Alanasana

11. *Parivrtta Alanasana* (Twisted High Lunge Pose)

12. Step forward to *Parivrtta Utkatasana* (Revolved Chair Pose)

13. *Utkatasana* (Chair Pose)

14. *Parivrtta Utkatasana* in opposite direction of step 12 (toward left side)

15. Step back to *Parivrtta Alanasana*

16. *Alanasana* with left foot forward

17. *Adho Mukha Svanasana* (Downward Facing Dog Pose)

18. Repeat steps 10–17 on other side, with left foot coming forward first.

19. *Balasana* (Child's Pose)

20. *Sukhasana* (Seated Meditation)

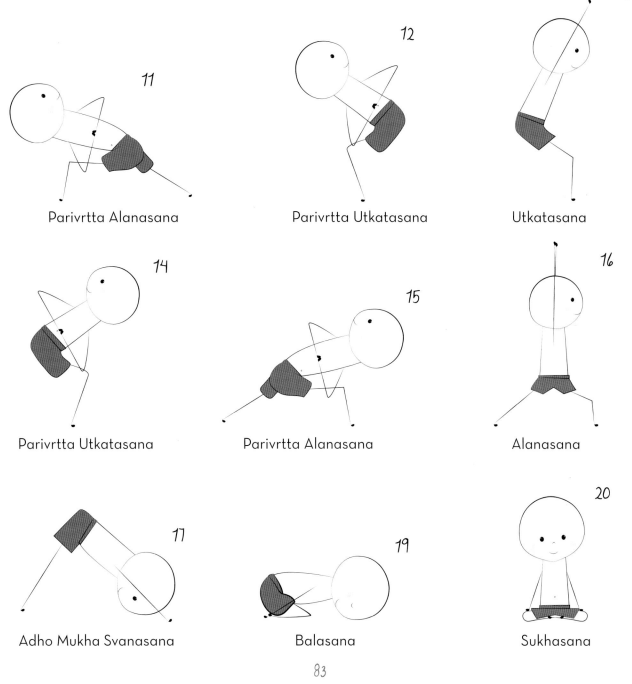

11 Parivrtta Alanasana

12 Parivrtta Utkatasana

13 Utkatasana

14 Parivrtta Utkatasana

15 Parivrtta Alanasana

16 Alanasana

17 Adho Mukha Svanasana

19 Balasana

20 Sukhasana

83

Yoga for Glowing, Gorgeous Skin

More than genetics and pizza grease, stress on your mind will stress out your skin. If you've ever looked at a row of yogis looking fresh and glowing as they exited the studio and wondered why you can't get that, well, you can. Yoga reduces stress levels and also aids in the natural processes of detoxification. My best advice for glowing, gorgeous skin? Get out your mat and find a fun flow that emphasizes detox and encourages you to sweat it out.

1. *Sukhasana* (Easy Pose)
2. *Nadi Shodana Pranayama* (Alternate Nostril Breath). Continue for 5-10 minutes.
3. *Ardha Matsyendrasana* (Half Seated Twist Pose). Repeat other direction.
4. *Tadasana* (Mountain Pose)
5. *Pavana Muktasana* (Standing Wind Relieving Pose)
6. *Vrksasana* (Tree Pose)
7. Repeat steps 5 and 6 on other side
8. *Trikonasana* (Triangle Pose)
9. *Parivrtta Trikonasana* (Revolved Triangle Pose)
10. Repeat steps 8 and 9 on other side
11. *Prasarita Padottanasana* (Wide-Legged Forward Bend)
12. *Parsvottanasana* (Intense Side Stretch Pose). Repeat on other side. Note: Focus on pulling the lower belly in to make space for the forward bend.

Turn to page 86 to complete sequence.

1 Sukhasana

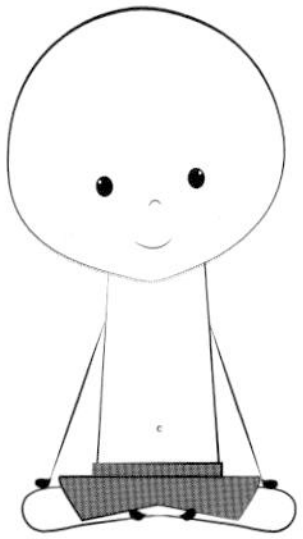

2 Pranayama

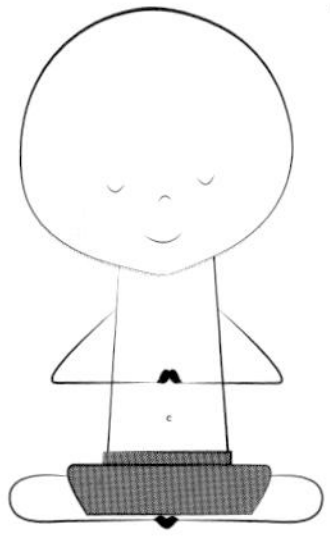

3 Ardha Matsyendrasana

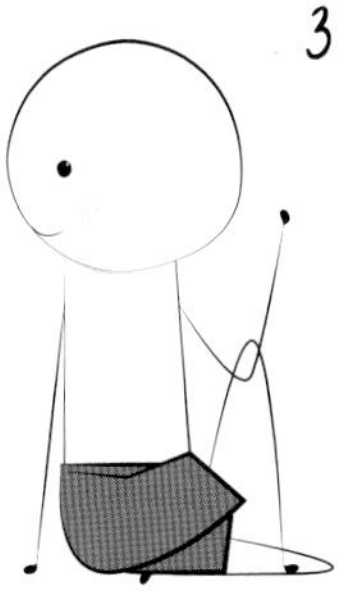

4 Tadasana

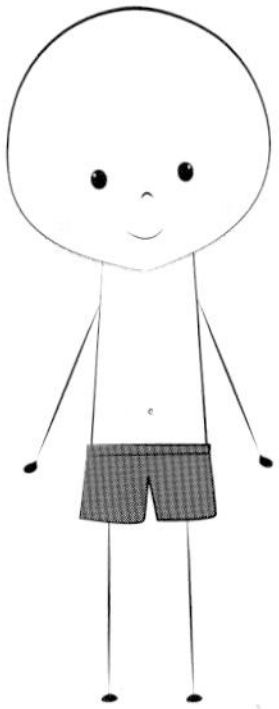

5 Pavana Muktasana

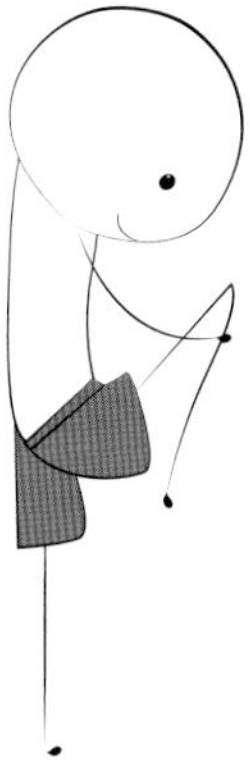

6 Vrksasana

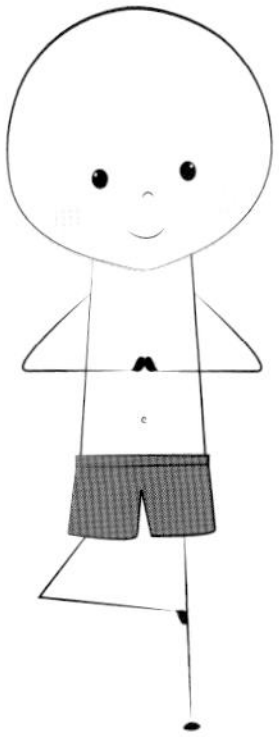

8 Trikonasana

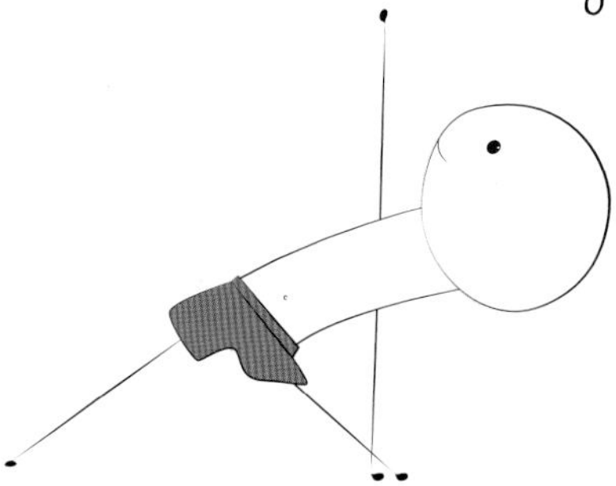

9 Parivrtta Trikonasana

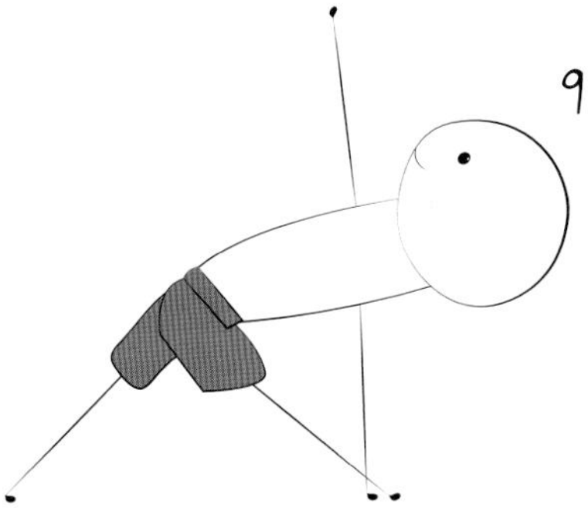

11 Prasarita Padottanasana

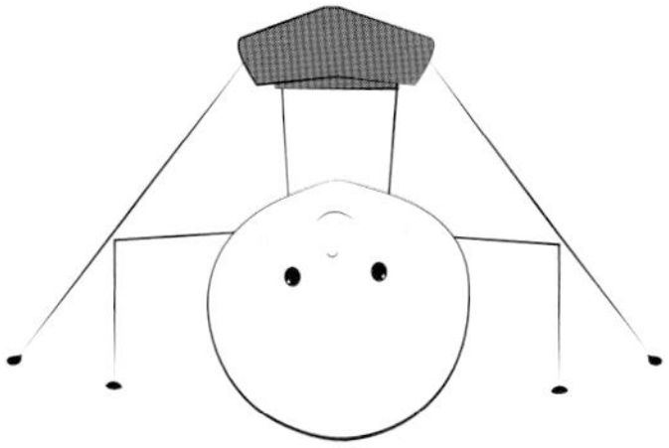

12 Parsvottanasana

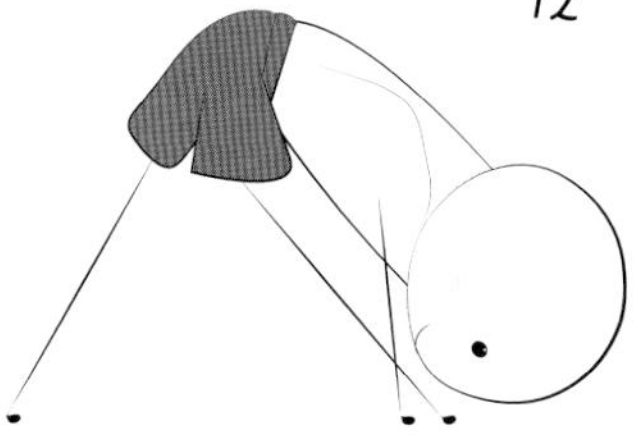

13. *Tadasana*

14. *Balasana* (Child's Pose)

15. Plank Pose on forearms

16. *Vasisthasana* (Side Plank Pose) on forearms. Repeat on other side.

17. Flow with breath between sides for 1–2 minutes

18. Sphinx

19. *Balasana*

20. *Supta Pavana Muktasana* (Reclined Wind Relieving Pose). Repeat on other side.

21. *Apanasana* (Knees to Chest on Back)

22. *Supta Matsyendrasana* (Reclined Twist Pose). Repeat on other side.

23. *Savasana* (Corpse Pose)

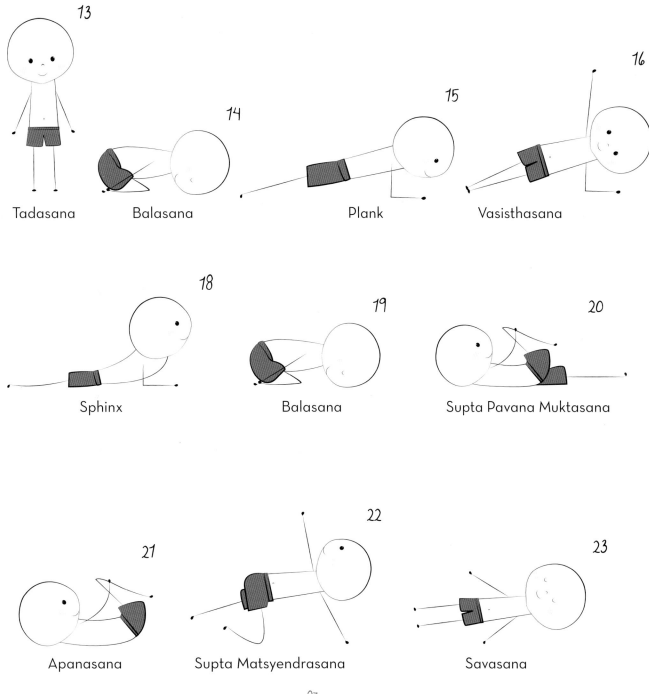

13
Tadasana

14
Balasana

15
Plank

16
Vasisthasana

18
Sphinx

19
Balasana

20
Supta Pavana Muktasana

21
Apanasana

22
Supta Matsyendrasana

23
Savasana

Heart-Opening Yoga Sequence

There are many ways in which we open our hearts. During long periods of traveling, I was invited into people's homes and lives everywhere I went. I came away from this experience overwhelmed with gratitude for the generosity of friends old and new. I feel a similar gratitude toward my yoga students. I am constantly in awe of how they allow themselves to be vulnerable and then appear fearless in the face of the unknown. If you choose to open your heart, getting on your mat day after day, no matter what, will help on that path.

1. *SUKHASANA* (Easy Pose)
2. Cat/Cow spine in seat
3. *PARIGHASANA* (Gate Pose)
4. Cat/Cow spine in Table Top
5. *PARIGHASANA* on other side
6. *USTRASANA* (Camel Pose)
7. *VAJRASANA* (Diamond Pose)
8. *ANAHATASANA* (Extended Puppy Dog Pose)
9. *ADHO MUKHA SVANASANA* (Downward Facing Dog Pose). Note: Press the heart forward here as you open the chest.
10. *TADASANA* (Mountain Pose)
11. *VIRABHADRASANA I* (Warrior I Pose)

TURN TO PAGE 90 TO COMPLETE SEQUENCE.

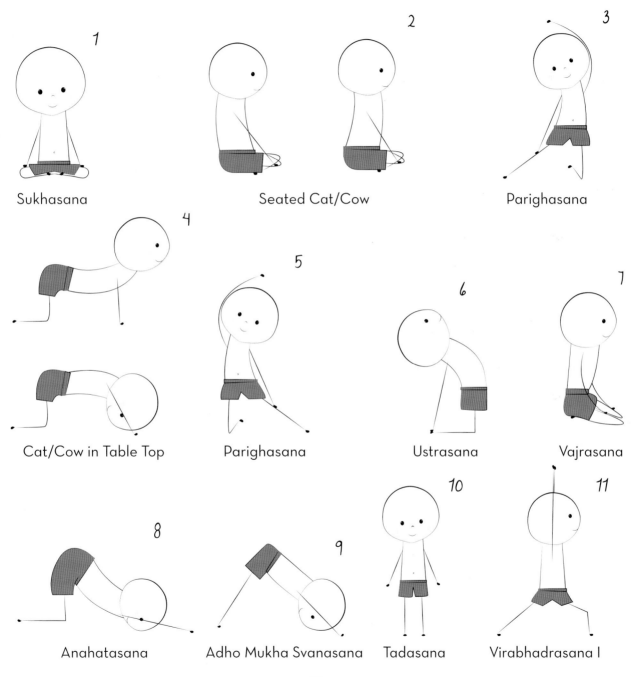

1 Sukhasana

2 Seated Cat/Cow

3 Parighasana

4 Cat/Cow in Table Top

5 Parighasana

6 Ustrasana

7 Vajrasana

8 Anahatasana

9 Adho Mukha Svanasana

10 Tadasana

11 Virabhadrasana I

12. *TADASANA*

13. *VIRABHADRASANA I* with other leg forward

14. *TADASANA*

15. *BADDHA VIRABHADRASANA* (Humble Warrior Pose)

16. Repeat steps 14 and 15 on other side

17. *SURYA NAMASKAR A* (Sun Salutations A), 4-6 times. Note: Feel as though the heart is literally leading you through each posture into the next. The upper chest is the first point of movement.

18. *SUKHASANA*

19. *NAVASANA* (Boat Pose)

20. *UPAVISHTA KONASANA* (Seated Wide Angle Forward Bend)

21. *ARDHA MATSYENDRASANA* (Half Seated Twist Pose). Repeat on other side.

22. *SETU BANDHASANA* (Bridge Pose)

23. *SAVASANA* (Corpse Pose)

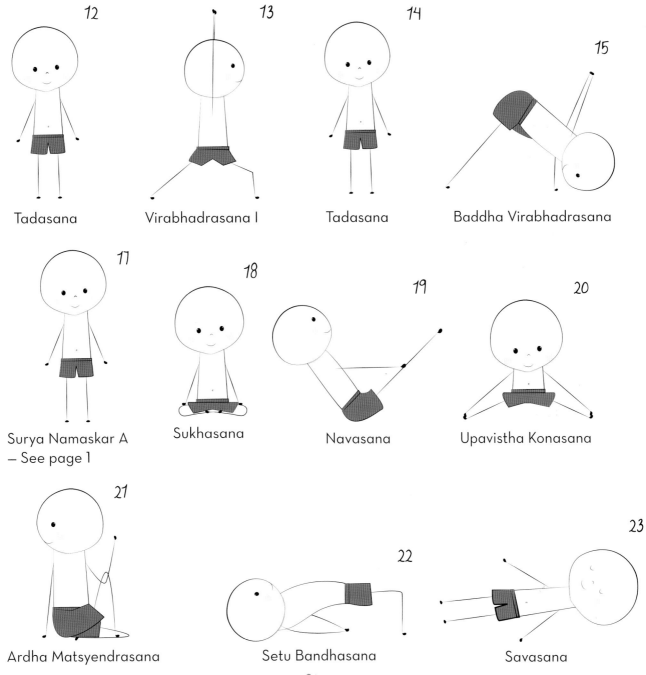

12 Tadasana

13 Virabhadrasana I

14 Tadasana

15 Baddha Virabhadrasana

17 Surya Namaskar A
— See page 1

18 Sukhasana

19 Navasana

20 Upavistha Konasana

21 Ardha Matsyendrasana

22 Setu Bandhasana

23 Savasana

Going with the Flow

I am not a patient person. Anyone who has spent more than five minutes with me can tell you that. Usually, I know where I want to go, and how I want to get there, and I don't really feel like waiting around while everyone else figures things out.

I'm working on it. By being patient with myself as I play with challenging poses, enjoying the journey of learning them instead of needing to "master" them immediately, I'm learning to let go a little bit. While I'm not quite there yet, flowing sequences help me on my way.

1. *BALASANA* (Child's Pose), 1–3 minutes
2. Table Top
3. *BHUJANGASANA* (Cobra Pose)
4. Table Top
5. *BALASANA*
6. Flow between steps 1–5. Repeat 5 times. Note: Use your upper body strength.
7. *ADHO MUKHA SVANASANA* (Downward Facing Dog Pose)
8. *UTTANASANA* (Standing Forward Fold)
9. *SURYA NAMASKAR A* (Sun Salutations A). Repeat 6 times.
10. *ADHO MUKHA SVANASANA*
11. *VIRABHADRASANA II* (Warrior II Pose)

TURN TO PAGE 94 TO COMPLETE SEQUENCE.

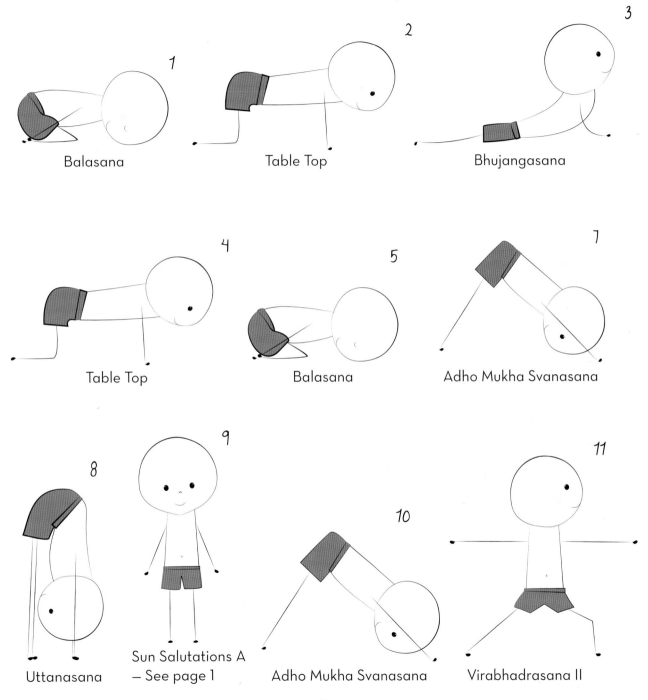

1 Balasana

2 Table Top

3 Bhujangasana

4 Table Top

5 Balasana

7 Adho Mukha Svanasana

8 Uttanasana

9 Sun Salutations A
— See page 1

10 Adho Mukha Svanasana

11 Virabhadrasana II

12. *UTHITTA PARSVAKONASANA* (Extended Side Angle Pose)

13. *VIPARITA VIRABHADRASANA* (Peaceful Warrior Pose)

14. Flow with your breath between steps 12 and 13

15. Repeat steps 10-14 on other side

16. *UTTANASANA* (Standing Forward Fold)

17. *UTKATASANA* (Chair Pose)

18. *PARIVRTTA UTKATASANA* (Revolved Chair Pose)

19. *UTKATASANA*

20. *PARIVRTTA UTKATASANA* twisting other way

21. Flow between steps 17 and 20. Repeat 3 times.

22. *UTTANASANA* (Standing Forward Fold)

23. *ADHO MUKHA SVANASANA*

24. *SUPTA KAPOTASANA* (Reclined Pigeon Pose). Repeat on other side.

25. *SAVASANA* (Corpse Pose)

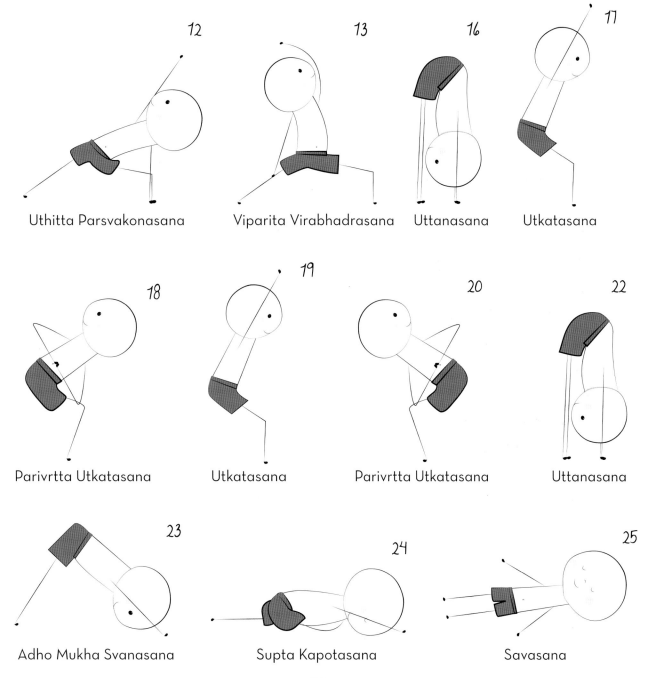

12 — Uthitta Parsvakonasana

13 — Viparita Virabhadrasana

16 — Uttanasana

17 — Utkatasana

18 — Parivrtta Utkatasana

19 — Utkatasana

20 — Parivrtta Utkatasana

22 — Uttanasana

23 — Adho Mukha Svanasana

24 — Supta Kapotasana

25 — Savasana

Strong and Powerful

Yoga for Head-to-Toe Toning

Hip Openers

My parents have a ginormous Great Dane named Achilles. He is a particularly special pup because he is somewhere between eleven and twelve years old, which is really, really old for a Great Dane. He is in splendid health. I think we can partially attribute Achilles's health to his magnificently flexible hips. In larger dogs, hip deterioration can lead to a plethora of other health issues and a shortened lifespan. (The average lifespan for Great Danes is around eight years.)

Hip health is just as important for us humans. Serious hip injuries in older adults (like fractures and breaks) may never heal. Just like Achilles, more mobility usually means improved health and a longer, happier life. So take good care of your hips with this hippy-happy sequence and watch every other part of your physical health improve, too.

1. *Ardha Ananda Balasana* (Half Happy Baby Pose). Repeat other side.

2. *Ananda Balasana* (Happy Baby Pose)

3. Cat/Cow spine in Table Top

4. *Adho Mukha Svanasana* (Downward Facing Dog Pose). Note: Lift one leg, bend at the knee, and draw circles with the knee. Repeat other side.

5. *Uttanasana* (Standing Forward Fold)

6. *Tadasana* (Mountain Pose)

7. *Vrksasana* (Tree Pose)

8. *Virabhadrasana III* (Warrior III Pose)

Turn to page 100 to continue sequence.

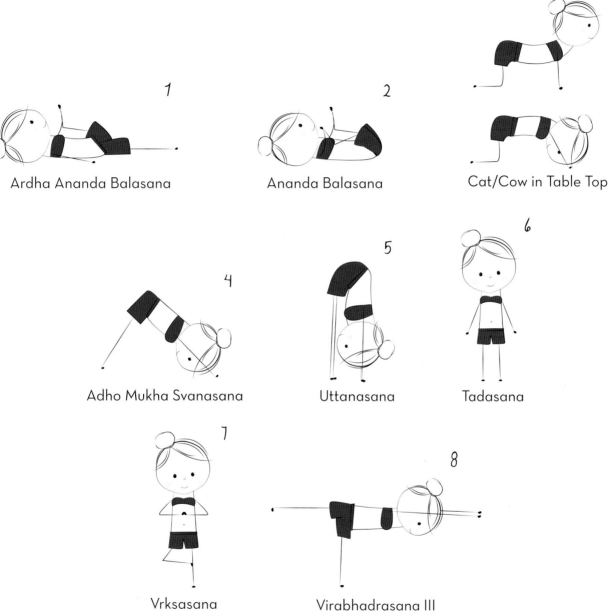

1

Ardha Ananda Balasana

2

Ananda Balasana

3

Cat/Cow in Table Top

4

Adho Mukha Svanasana

5

Uttanasana

6

Tadasana

7

Vrksasana

8

Virabhadrasana III

9. *Virabhadrasana II* (Warrior II Pose)

10. *Deviasana* (Goddess Pose or Horse Stance). Note: Hold for 10 cycles of breath, gently pulsing into and out of the pose with each exhale and inhale.

11. *Virabhadrasana II*

12. *Alanasana* (High Lunge Pose)

13. *Baddha Virabhadrasana* (Humble Warrior Pose)

14. *Utthan Pristasana* (Lizard Pose)

15. Plank Pose

16. *Vasisthasana* (Side Plank Pose). Note: Come onto the hand that is on same side as foot that had been forward during the standing poses.

Turn to page 102 to complete sequence.

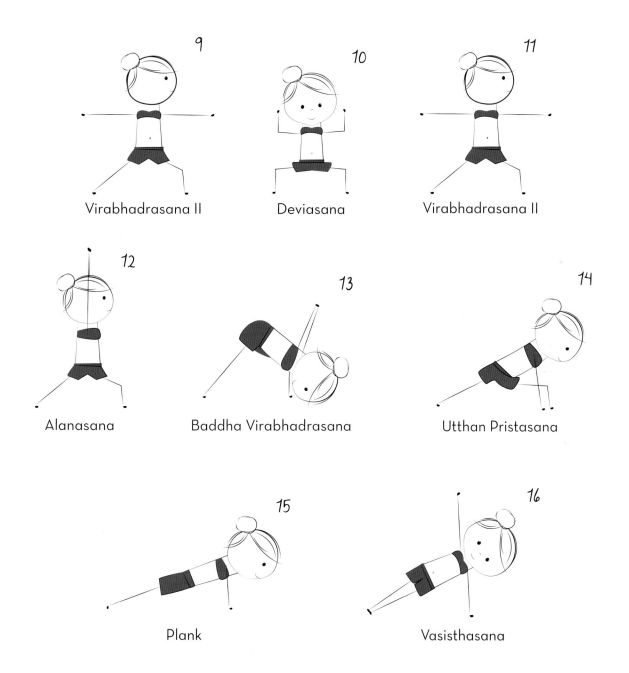

9
Virabhadrasana II

10
Deviasana

11
Virabhadrasana II

12
Alanasana

13
Baddha Virabhadrasana

14
Utthan Pristasana

15
Plank

16
Vasisthasana

17. Plank Pose

18. *Urdhva Mukha Svanasana* (Upward Facing Dog Pose)

19. *Adho Mukha Svanasana*

20. Repeat steps 6-19 on other side

21. *Bhekasana* (Frog Pose). Hold for 2 minutes.

22. *Setu Bandhasana* (Bridge Pose). Hold for 2 minutes.

23. *Supta Matsyendrasana* (Reclined Twist Pose). Repeat other side.

24. *Savasana* (Corpse Pose)

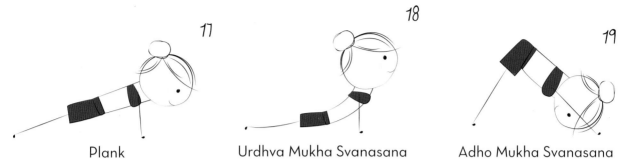

17
Plank

18
Urdhva Mukha Svanasana

19
Adho Mukha Svanasana

21
Bhekasana

22
Setu Bandhasana

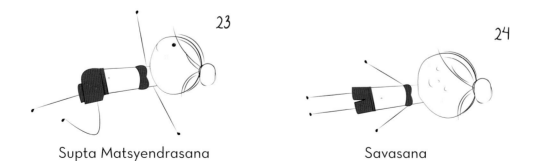

23
Supta Matsyendrasana

24
Savasana

Hard Core Yoga Sequence

All of my yoga sequences are Hard Core. By that, I mean I ask a lot of my students: flow, breath, and attention. In this sequence, however, I specifically intend for these poses to strengthen your abdominal muscles. I teach more "Core" classes in the winter (it's a good way to heat up quickly), but that doesn't mean it's not fun to practice them all year round. They are always good to help with digestion, decrease lower back pain (if done correctly), and help with posture. With this practice, you can be Hard Core every day.

1. *BALASANA* (Child's Pose)
2. *ADHO MUKHA SVANASANA* (Downward Facing Dog Pose)
3. Plank Pose. Hold for 1-2 minutes.
4. *BALASANA*
5. *NAVASANA* (Boat Pose)
6. *BALASANA*
7. *NAVASANA*
8. Cat/Cow spine in Table Top

TURN TO PAGE 106 TO CONTINUE SEQUENCE.

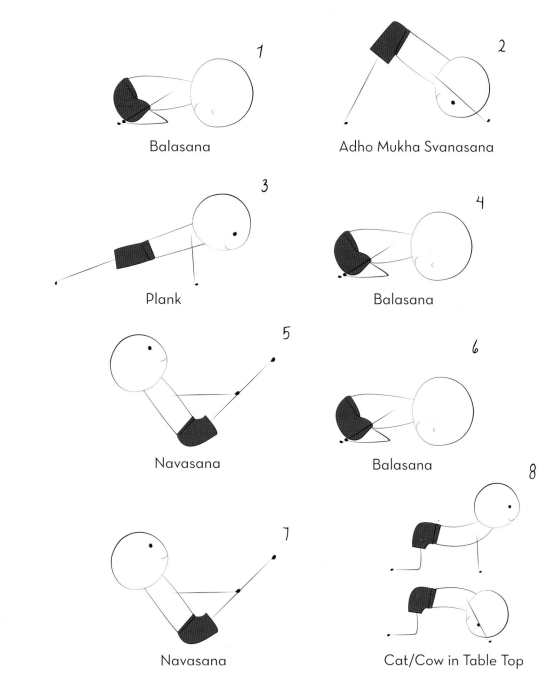

1 Balasana

2 Adho Mukha Svanasana

3 Plank

4 Balasana

5 Navasana

6 Balasana

7 Navasana

8 Cat/Cow in Table Top

9. *Adho Mukha Svanasana*

10. Plank Pose

11. *Vasisthasana* (Side Plank Pose). Hold for 1 minute. Repeat other side.

12. *Adho Mukha Svanasana*

13. *Tadasana* (Mountain Pose)

14. *Garundasana* (Eagle Pose). Repeat other side.

Turn to page 108 to continue sequence.

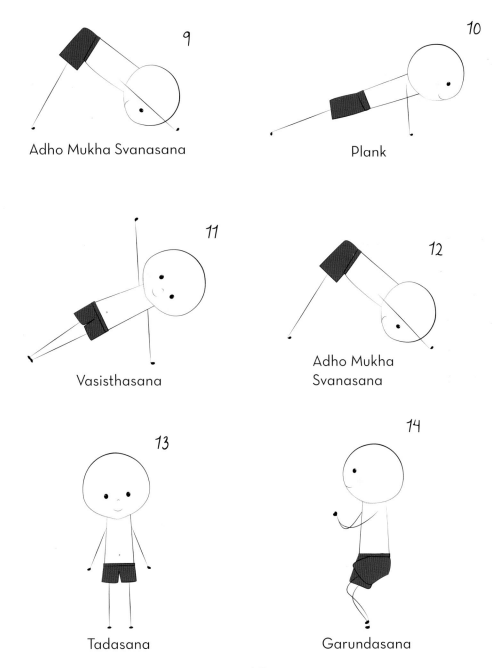

9 Adho Mukha Svanasana

10 Plank

11 Vasisthasana

12 Adho Mukha Svanasana

13 Tadasana

14 Garundasana

15. *Natarajasana* (Dancer's Pose). Repeat other side.

16. *Tadasana*

17. *Pavana Muktasana* (Standing Wind Relieving Pose)

18. *Virabhadrasana III* (Warrior III Pose)

19. *Virabhadrasana I* (Warrior I Pose)

20. *Virabhadrasana II* (Warrior II Pose)

21. *Trikonasana* (Triangle Pose)

Turn to page 110 to complete sequence.

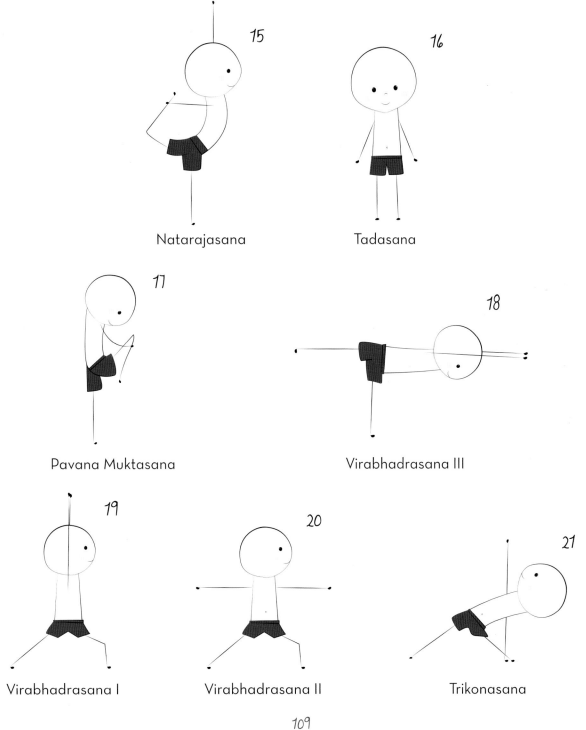

15 Natarajasana

16 Tadasana

17 Pavana Muktasana

18 Virabhadrasana III

19 Virabhadrasana I

20 Virabhadrasana II

21 Trikonasana

22. *VIRABHADRASANA II*

23. Repeat steps 16–22 on other side

24. *CHATURANGA DANDASANA* (Four Limbed Staff Pose)

25. *URDHVA MUKHA SVANASANA* (Upward Facing Dog Pose)

26. *ADHO MUKHA SVANASANA*

27. *SETU BANDHASANA* (Bridge Pose)

28. *SUPTA MATSYENDRASANA* (Reclined Twist Pose). Repeat other side.

29. *SAVASANA* (Corpse Pose)

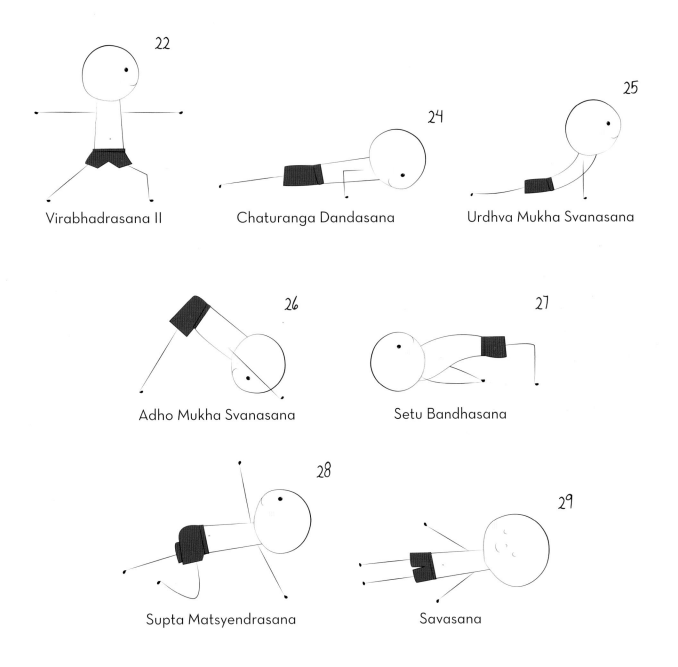

22 Virabhadrasana II

24 Chaturanga Dandasana

25 Urdhva Mukha Svanasana

26 Adho Mukha Svanasana

27 Setu Bandhasana

28 Supta Matsyendrasana

29 Savasana

Leg Strengtheners

I hate running. I know some people say it's meditation in motion, and good for them. For folks like me, we have to turn to our yoga practice to de-jiggle our thighs. Good thing there is a huge range of poses to strengthen every part of our legs from ankles (balancing poses) to quads and hamstrings (hello, Chair Pose!). In this sequence, you will find poses to make the legs stronger and more flexible, too. Go ahead and throw out your running shoes, and step onto your yoga mat!

1. *SAVASANA* (Corpse Pose)
2. *SETU BANDHASANA* (Bridge Pose)
3. *APANASANA* (Knees to Chest on Back)
4. *NAVASANA* (Boat Pose). Note: Really engage the leg muscles here to make it easier on the core.
5. *BALASANA* (Child's Pose)
6. Plank Pose
7. *CHATURANGA DANDASANA* (Four Limbed Staff Pose)
8. *URDHVA MUKHA SVANASANA* (Upward Facing Dog Pose)

TURN TO PAGE 114 TO CONTINUE SEQUENCE.

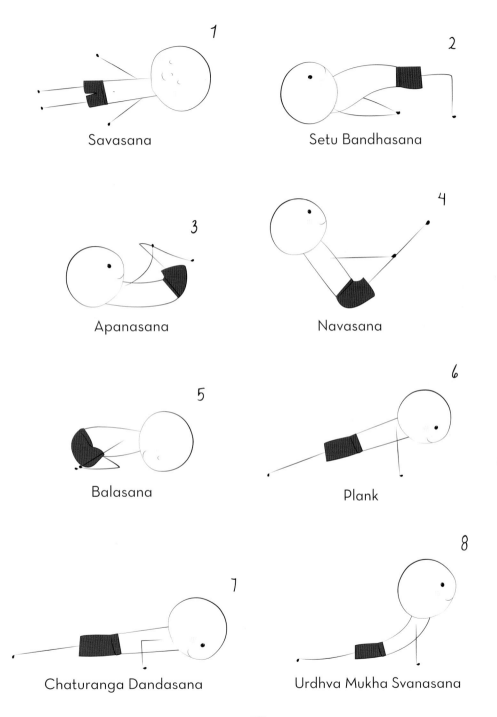

1
Savasana

2
Setu Bandhasana

3
Apanasana

4
Navasana

5
Balasana

6
Plank

7
Chaturanga Dandasana

8
Urdhva Mukha Svanasana

9. *Adho Mukha Svanasana* (Downward Facing Dog Pose)

10. Repeat steps 5–9 five times

11. *Tadasana* (Mountain Pose)

12. *Vrksasana* (Tree Pose). Repeat other side.

13. *Virabhadrasana III* (Warrior III Pose). Repeat other side.

14. *Natarajasana* (Dancer's Pose). Repeat other side.

15. *Virabhadrasana I* (Warrior I Pose)

16. *Virabhadrasana II* (Warrior II Pose)

17. *Trikonanasana* (Triangle Pose)

18. Repeat steps 15–17 on other side

Turn to page 116 to complete sequence.

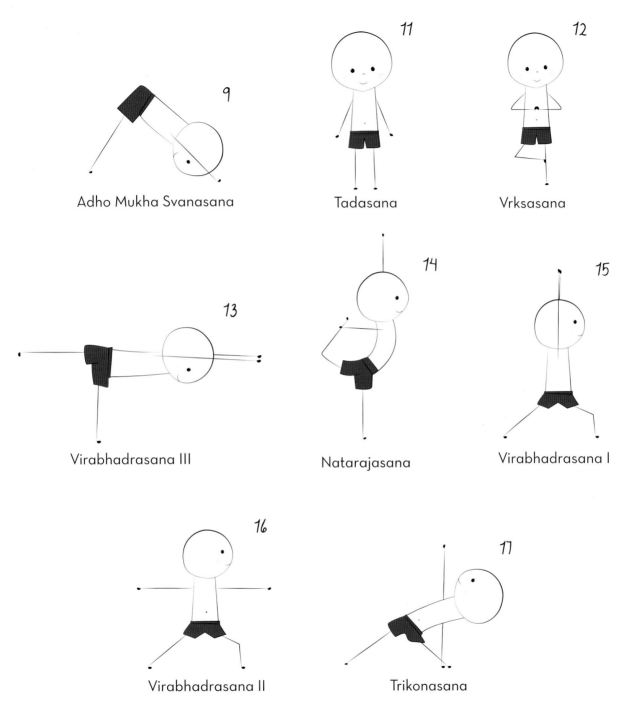

9 Adho Mukha Svanasana

11 Tadasana

12 Vrksasana

13 Virabhadrasana III

14 Natarajasana

15 Virabhadrasana I

16 Virabhadrasana II

17 Trikonasana

115

19. *Utkatasana* (Chair Pose). Note: Hold 1–2 minutes, pulsing deeper into the pose with every exhale, coming out a little with every inhale.

20. *Uttanasana* (Standing Forward Fold)

21. *Paschimottanasana* (Seated Forward Fold)

22. *Upavishta Konasana* (Seated Wide Angle Forward Bend)

23. *Supta Padangustasana* (Reclined Big Toe Pose)

24. *Supta Trivikramasana* (Reclined Vishnu Pose)

25. *Urdhva Mukha Paschimottanasana* (Upward Facing Fold Pose)

26. Repeat steps 23–25 on other side

27. *Savasana* (Corpse Pose)

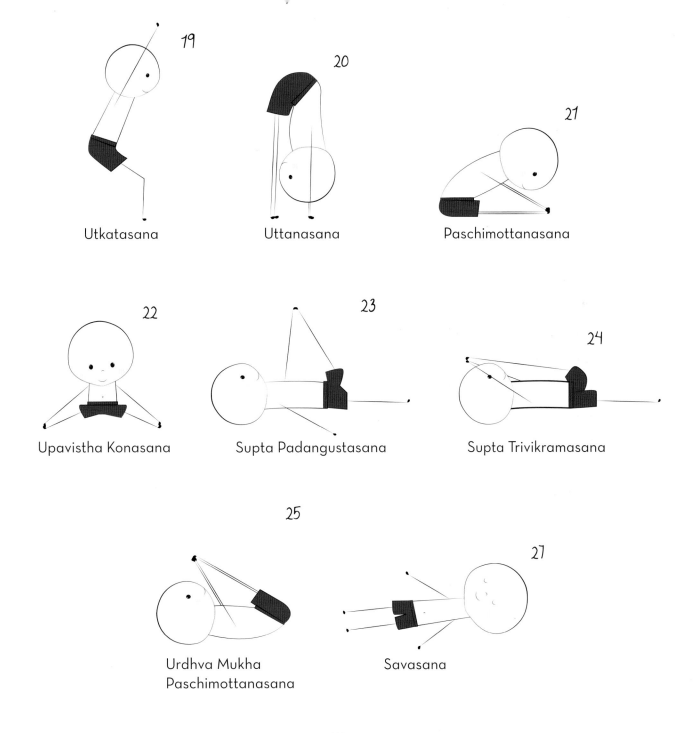

19
Utkatasana

20
Uttanasana

21
Paschimottanasana

22
Upavistha Konasana

23
Supta Padangustasana

24
Supta Trivikramasana

25
Urdhva Mukha
Paschimottanasana

27
Savasana

Superhero Arms

Men, anatomically, tend to have stronger upper bodies. It can be frustrating to work on a pose for months, just to see a dude, on his first try, muscle his way through. Sure, the gift is in the journey. It's also not a bad idea for the ladies to work on upper-body strength and develop their bodies (along with their practice) more evenly.

If you feel like your arms are giving out and not allowing you to maintain the integrity of the poses, come into Child's Pose. Trying to work around overtired arms can lead to injuries, because who knows what will end up overcompensating. Often the first indicator that we are practicing at a more physically challenging level than we are prepared for is that the breath begins to quicken and becomes erratic. Again, if this is the case, take a break from the sequence. It will still be there for you to come back to.

1. *Vajrasana* (Diamond Pose)
2. Cat/Cow spine in Table Top
3. Plank Pose
4. *Chaturanga Dandasana* (Four Limbed Staff Pose)
5. Plank Pose
6. *Chaturanga Dandasana*. Note: Count to ten in your mind, slowly lowering yourself to your belly as you count down.
7. *Salabhasana* (Locust Pose)
8. *Chaturanga Dandasana*

Turn to page 120 to continue sequence.

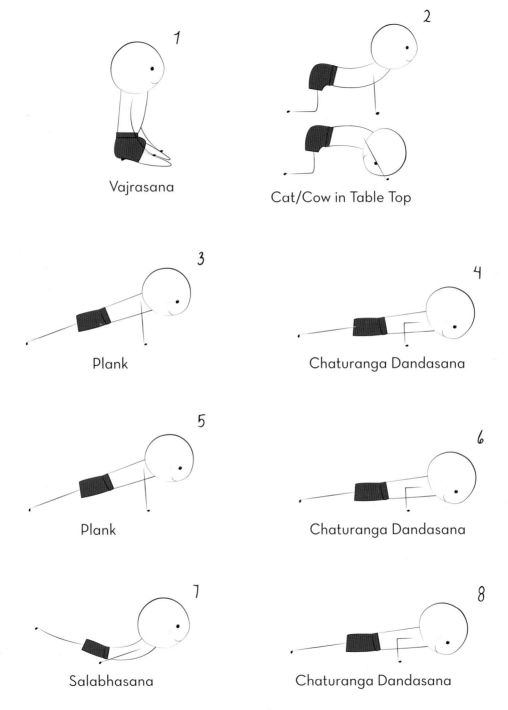

1 Vajrasana

2 Cat/Cow in Table Top

3 Plank

4 Chaturanga Dandasana

5 Plank

6 Chaturanga Dandasana

7 Salabhasana

8 Chaturanga Dandasana

9. Plank Pose

10. *Adho Mukha Svanasana* (Downward Facing Dog Pose)

11. *Garundasana* (Eagle Pose)

12. *Virabhadrasana I* (Warrior I Pose)

13. *Virabhadrasana II* (Warrior II Pose)

14. Repeat steps 10–13 on other side

15. *Adho Mukha Svanasana*

16. *Urdhva Mukha Svanasana* (Upward Facing Dog Pose)

17. *Bhujangasana* (Cobra Pose). Note: After Bhujangasana, release onto the belly. Counting to ten in your mind, slowly lift yourself up to Plank Pose.

Turn to page 122 to complete sequence.

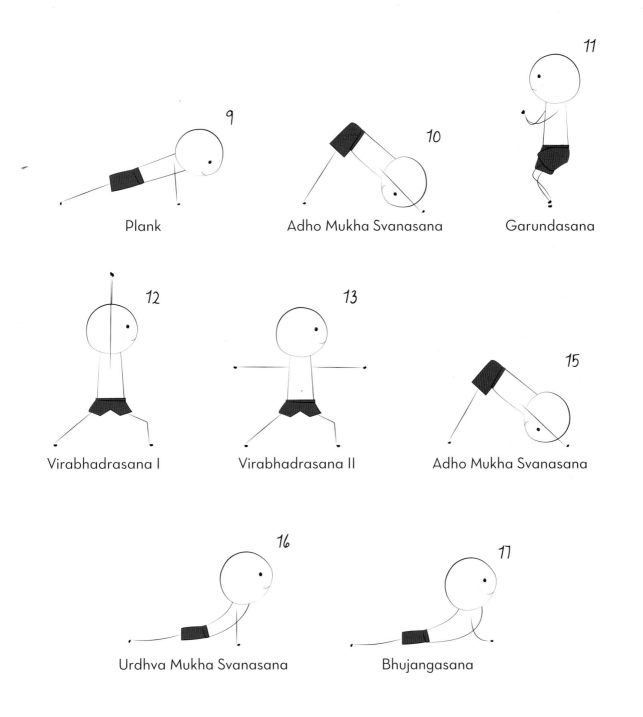

9
Plank

10
Adho Mukha Svanasana

11
Garundasana

12
Virabhadrasana I

13
Virabhadrasana II

15
Adho Mukha Svanasana

16
Urdhva Mukha Svanasana

17
Bhujangasana

18. Plank Pose

19. *Adho Mukha Svanasana*

20. *Vasisthasana* (Side Plank Pose). Repeat other side.

21. *Adho Mukha Svanasana*

22. *Balasana* (Child's Pose)

23. *Dhanurasana* (Bow Pose)

24. *Balasana*

25. *Gomukhasana* (Cow Face Pose). Repeat other side.

26. *Savasana* (Corpse Pose)

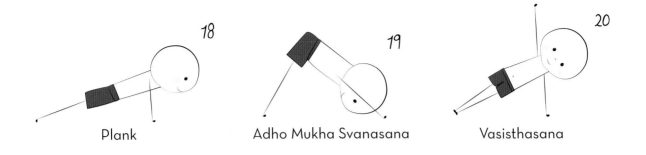

Plank

Adho Mukha Svanasana

Vasisthasana

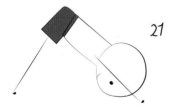

Adho Mukha Svanasana

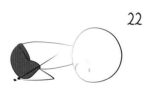

Balasana

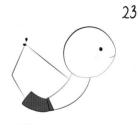

Dhanurasana

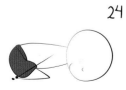

Balasana

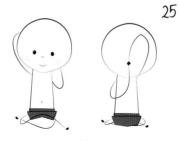

Gomukhasana

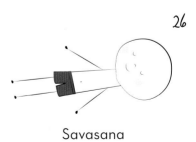

Savasana

Tushy Toners

Gravity has all sorts of benefits—like allowing human life on Earth. That being said, gravity can have some less-than-ideal effects on our physical bodies. Our spines compress, our skin sags, and, yes, our booties move southward. Good thing yoga laughs in the face of gravity. Just take the time to practice this sequence once a week, and you can laugh at gravity, too.

1. *Tadasana* (Mountain Pose)
2. *Utkatasana* (Chair Pose)
3. *Alanasana* (High Lunge Pose)
4. *Parivrtta Alanasana* (Twisted High Lunge Pose)
5. *Virabhadrasana II* (Warrior II Pose)
6. *Trikonasana* (Triangle Pose)
7. *Parsvottanasana* (Intense Side Stretch Pose)
8. *Parivrtta Trikonasana* (Revolved Triangle Pose)

Turn to page 126 to continue sequence.

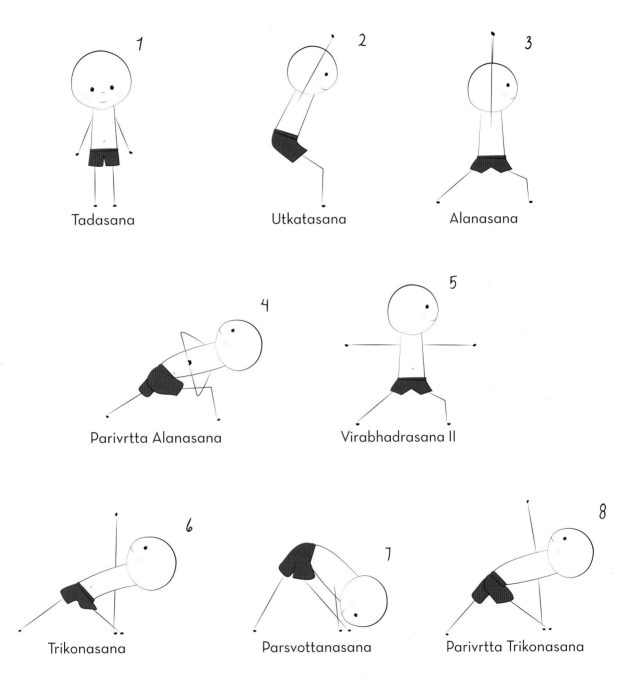

1 Tadasana

2 Utkatasana

3 Alanasana

4 Parivrtta Alanasana

5 Virabhadrasana II

6 Trikonasana

7 Parsvottanasana

8 Parivrtta Trikonasana

9. *Tadasana*

10. Repeat steps 2-9 on other side

11. *Utkatasana*

12. *Parivrtta Utkatasana* (Revolved Chair Pose). Repeat other side.

13. *Tadasana*

14. *Virabhadrasana III* (Warrior III Pose)

15. *Ardha Chandrasana* (Balancing Half Moon Pose)

16. *Parivrtta Ardha Chandrasana* (Revolved Balancing Half Moon Pose)

17. *Virabhadrasana III*

Turn to page 128 to complete sequence.

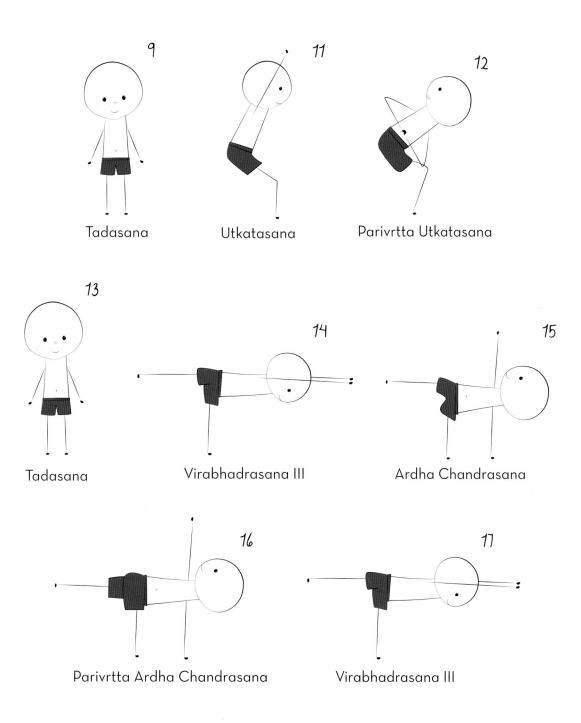

9
Tadasana

11
Utkatasana

12
Parivrtta Utkatasana

13
Tadasana

14
Virabhadrasana III

15
Ardha Chandrasana

16
Parivrtta Ardha Chandrasana

17
Virabhadrasana III

18. *ALANASANA* (High Lunge Pose)

19. Plank Pose on forearms. Hold for 1–2 minutes.

20. *BALASANA* (Child's Pose)

21. *ADHO MUKHA SVANASANA* (Downward Facing Dog Pose)

22. Repeat steps 11–20 on other side

23. *ARDHA MATSYENDRASANA* (Half Seated Twist Pose). Repeat other side.

24. *HALASANA* (Plow Pose)

25. *PASCHIMOTTANASANA* (Seated Forward Fold)

26. *SAVASANA* (Corpse Pose)

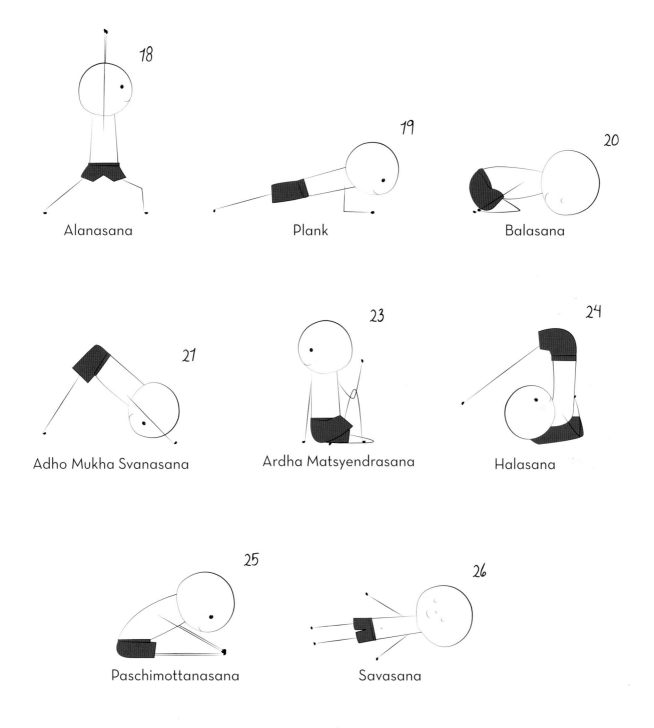

18

Alanasana

19

Plank

20

Balasana

21

Adho Mukha Svanasana

23

Ardha Matsyendrasana

24

Halasana

25

Paschimottanasana

26

Savasana

The Great Outdoors

After Activities Yoga

Yoga for Gardeners

I used to be on the Board of Directors for my local community garden, but here's my confession: sometimes, all of that forward folding, raking, and hoeing just makes my body feel exhausted and totally out of alignment. Some days, I'd be just as happy buying my greens from the farmers' market. For all of you yogis who can't be stopped from playing in the dirt, here's a restorative yoga sequence to help uncrunch your backs and even out the sides of the body.

1. *Tadasana* (Mountain Pose)
2. *Garundasana* (Eagle Pose). Repeat on other side.
3. *Anjaneyasana* (Knee-down Lunge Pose). Repeat on other side.
4. *Balasana* (Child's Pose). Hold for 3-5 minutes with a pillow under your torso.
5. *Setu Bandhasana* (Bridge Pose)
6. *Supta Baddha Konasana* (Reclined Bound Angle Pose). Hold for 3-5 minutes.
7. *Supta Matsyendrasana* (Reclined Twist Pose). Hold for 3-5 minutes on each side.
8. *Viparita Karani* (Legs up the Wall Pose)
9. *Savasana* (Corpse Pose)

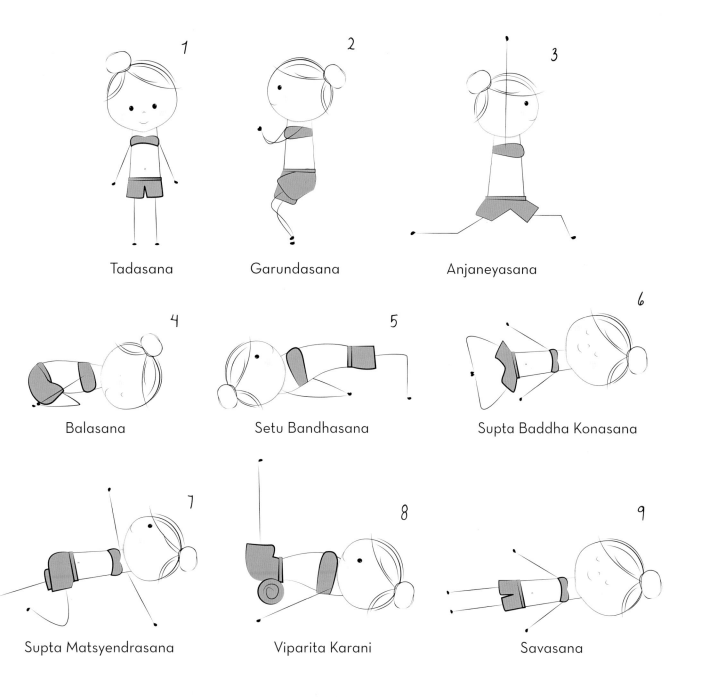

1 Tadasana

2 Garundasana

3 Anjaneyasana

4 Balasana

5 Setu Bandhasana

6 Supta Baddha Konasana

7 Supta Matsyendrasana

8 Viparita Karani

9 Savasana

Yoga for Cyclists

During the time I traveled around the United States looking for a place to live, I biked from Ithaca, New York, to Ann Arbor, Michigan. A few weeks later, I biked a meandering path across Iowa. After spending that much time in the saddle, I feel pretty confident I know a few tips and tricks for a good postcycling stretch. Depending on how long you were cycling, you might want to hold poses for more or less time and moderate how deeply you go into the poses.

1. *SUKHASANA* (Easy Pose)

2. *JANU SIRSASANA* (Head to Knee Pose)

3. *PARIVRTTA JANU SIRSASANA* (Revolved Head to Knee Pose)

4. *UPAVISTHA KONASANA* (Seated Wide Angle)

5. Repeat steps 2–4 on other side

6. *BADDHA KONASANA* (Bound Angle Pose)

7. *ADHO MUKHA SVANASANA* (Downward Facing Dog Pose). Take the legs wider than usual.

8. *PRASARITA PADOTTANASANA* (Wide-Legged Forward Bend)

9. *PARSVOTTANASANA* (Intense Side Stretch Pose)

TURN TO PAGE 136 TO COMPLETE SEQUENCE.

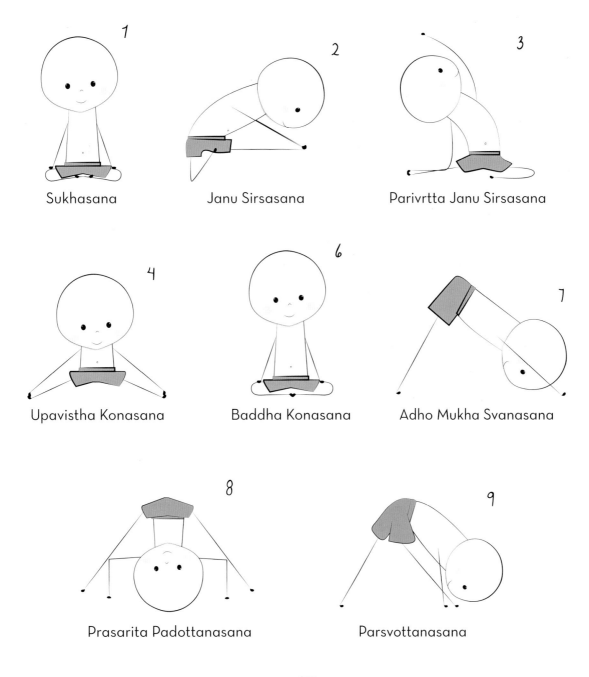

1 Sukhasana

2 Janu Sirsasana

3 Parivrtta Janu Sirsasana

4 Upavistha Konasana

6 Baddha Konasana

7 Adho Mukha Svanasana

8 Prasarita Padottanasana

9 Parsvottanasana

10. *Virabhadrasana I* (Warrior I Pose)

11. *Virabhadrasana II* (Warrior II Pose)

12. *Trikonasana* (Triangle Pose)

13. Repeat steps 7–12 on other side

14. *Adho Mukha Svanasana* (Downward Facing Dog Pose)

15. *Ardha Hanumanasana* (Half Split Pose)

16. Repeat steps 14 and 15 with other leg

17. *Tarasana* (Star Pose)

18. *Supta Matsyendrasana* (Reclined Twist Pose). Repeat on other side.

19. *Savasana* (Corpse Pose)

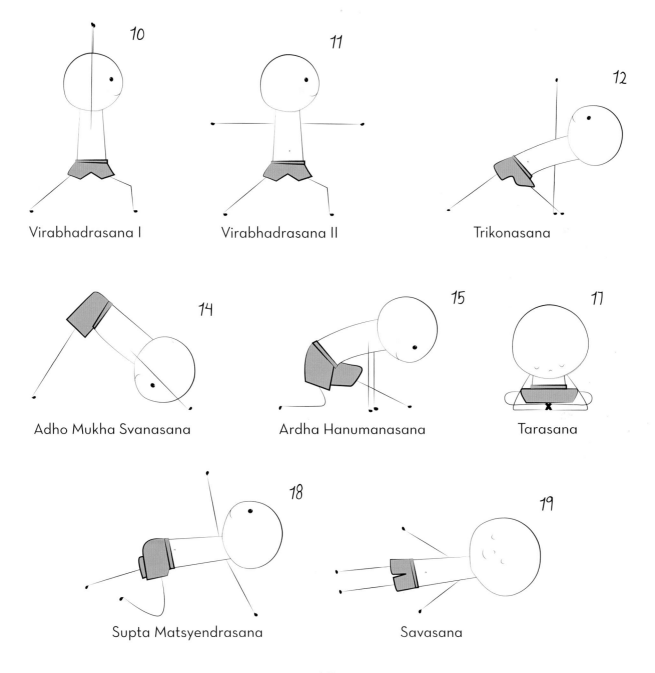

10 Virabhadrasana I

11 Virabhadrasana II

12 Trikonasana

14 Adho Mukha Svanasana

15 Ardha Hanumanasana

17 Tarasana

18 Supta Matsyendrasana

19 Savasana

Yoga after Taking a Hike

The word VACATION brings many things to mind: lounging on the beach, making your way through popular novels, drinking and eating copious amounts of fruit, etc. Somehow, however, on every vacation I find myself taking massive hikes and thinking, "Is this my vacation?"

Yup, this is my vacation. I love hiking, and lounging on the beach feels so much more earned after a full week of treks. Sometimes, however, hikes do some serious damage to my shins. If I want to be able to enjoy the rest of my time on vacation without hobbling around, I always turn to yoga. No matter if you're on vacation or just tromping around in the woods behind your house, this sequence will keep you on your feet after a great hike.

1. Sphinx Pose
2. *BHUJANGASANA* (Cobra Pose). Lift and lower slowly, waving the torso to come gently into Cobra.
3. *SUPTA KAPOTASANA* (Reclined Pigeon Pose). Repeat on other side.
4. *SUPTA PADANGUSTASANA* (Reclined Big Toe Pose)
5. *SUPTA TRIVIKRAMASANA* (Reclined Vishnu Pose)
6. *URDHVA MUKHA PASCHIMOTTANASANA* (Upward Facing Fold Pose)
7. Repeat steps 4-6 with other leg
8. *APANASANA* (Knees to Chest on Back)
9. *ARDHA MATSYENDRASANA* (Half Seated Twist Pose). Repeat on other side.
10. *TADASANA* (Mountain Pose)

TURN TO PAGE 140 TO COMPLETE SEQUENCE.

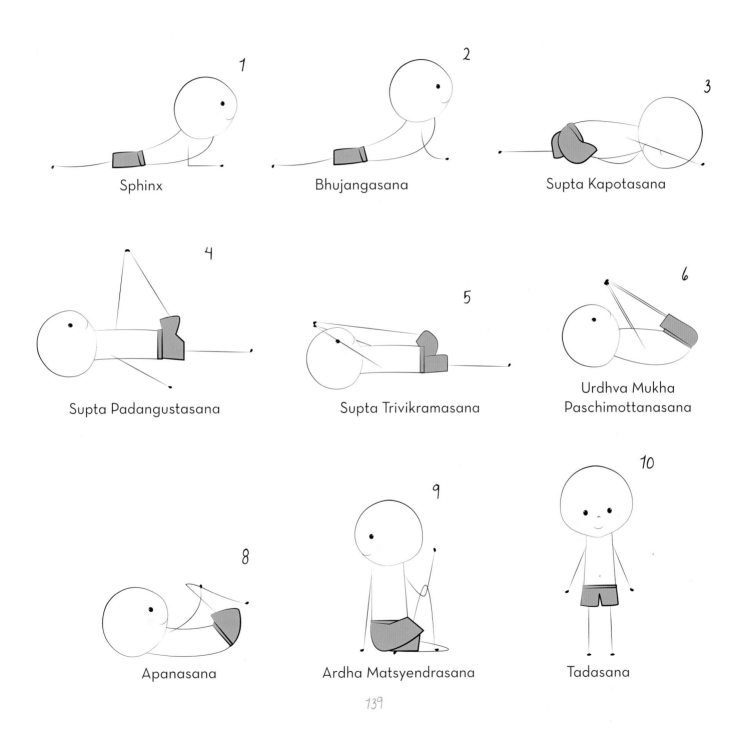

1 Sphinx

2 Bhujangasana

3 Supta Kapotasana

4 Supta Padangustasana

5 Supta Trivikramasana

6 Urdhva Mukha Paschimottanasana

8 Apanasana

9 Ardha Matsyendrasana

10 Tadasana

11. *UTTANASANA* (Standing Forward Fold). Hold 2–3 minutes.

12. *URDHVA HASTASANA* (Upward Hands Pose)

13. *PARSVOTTANASANA* (Intense Side Stretch Pose). Repeat on other side.

14. *NATARAJASANA* (Dancer's Pose). Repeat on other side.

15. *PRASARITA PADOTTANASANA* (Wide-Legged Forward Bend). Note: Interlock fingers behind back to get a back and shoulder stretch as well.

16. *URDHVA HASTASANA*

17. *MALASANA* (Seated Squat Pose). Hold for 1–2 minutes.

18. *JANU SIRSASANA* (Head to Knee Pose). Repeat on other side.

19. *SUPTA VIRASANA* (Reclined Heroes Pose)

20. *SAVASANA* (Corpse Pose)

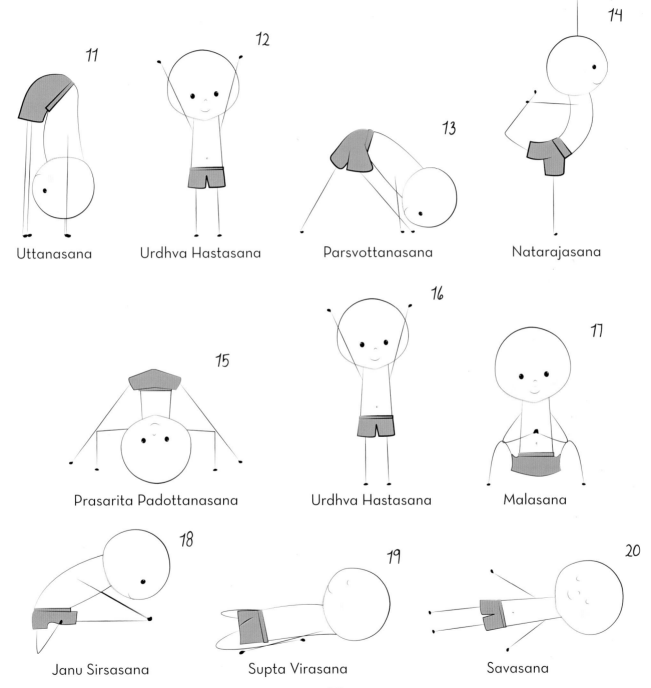

11 Uttanasana

12 Urdhva Hastasana

13 Parsvottanasana

14 Natarajasana

15 Prasarita Padottanasana

16 Urdhva Hastasana

17 Malasana

18 Janu Sirsasana

19 Supta Virasana

20 Savasana

Yoga for Runners

Remember how I said I really enjoy taking hikes? And how I biked across a few states? Maybe it somehow appears I spend every waking moment doing yoga? If I'm being honest with myself, I do all this physical activity just so I have an excuse to never, ever go on a run. I hate running with a passion unequaled. That being said, I know other people are quite fond of it (of course, they are delusional). The main difference between **Yoga after a Hike** and **Yoga for Runners** is the attention to healing sore knees. Especially if you run on the pavement, take the time to practice yoga and save yourself knee aches later on.

1. *Savasana* (Corpse Pose)
2. *Supta Padangustasana* (Reclined Big Toe Pose)
3. *Supta Trivikramasana* (Reclined Vishnu Pose)
4. *Urdhva Mukha Paschimottanasana* (Upward Facing Fold Pose)
5. Repeat steps 2–4 on other side
6. *Supta Pavana Muktasana* (Reclined Wind Relieving Pose). Repeat on other side.
7. *Setu Bandhasana* (Bridge Pose)
8. *Vajrasana* (Diamond Pose)
9. *Gomukhasana* (Cow Face Pose). Repeat on other side.
10. *Supta Virasana* (Reclined Heroes Pose)

Turn to page 144 to complete sequence.

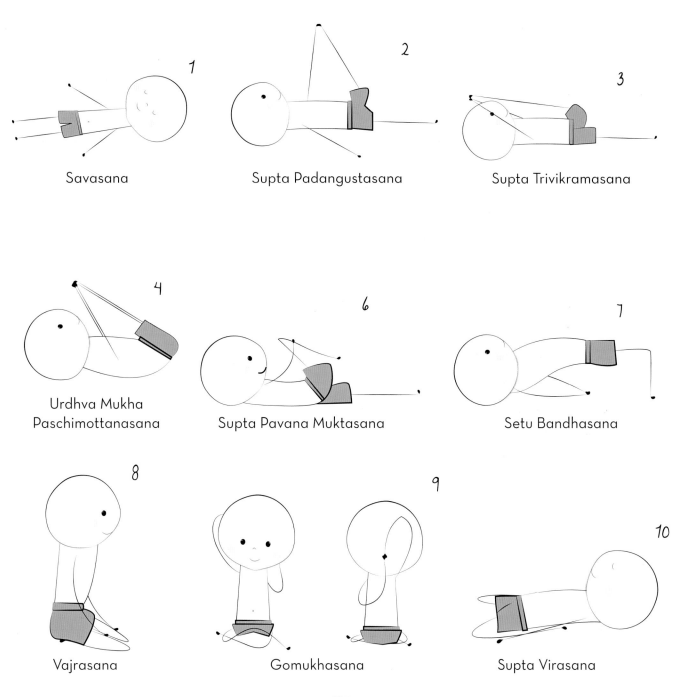

1 Savasana

2 Supta Padangustasana

3 Supta Trivikramasana

4 Urdhva Mukha Paschimottanasana

6 Supta Pavana Muktasana

7 Setu Bandhasana

8 Vajrasana

9 Gomukhasana

10 Supta Virasana

11.   *Ardha Matsyendrasana* (Half Seated Twist Pose). Repeat on other side.

12.   *Supta Kapotasana* (Reclined Pigeon Pose). Repeat on other side.

13.   *Adho Mukha Svanasana* (Downward Facing Dog Pose)

14.   *Parsvottanasana* (Intense Side Stretch Pose)

15.   Repeat steps 13 and 14 on other side

16.   *Adho Mukha Svanasana*

17.   *Anjaneyasana* (Knee-down Lunge Pose)

18.   *Ardha Hanumanasana* (Half Split Pose)

19.   Cat/Cow spine in Table Top

20.   Repeat steps 16-19 on other side

21.   *Savasana* (Corpse Pose)

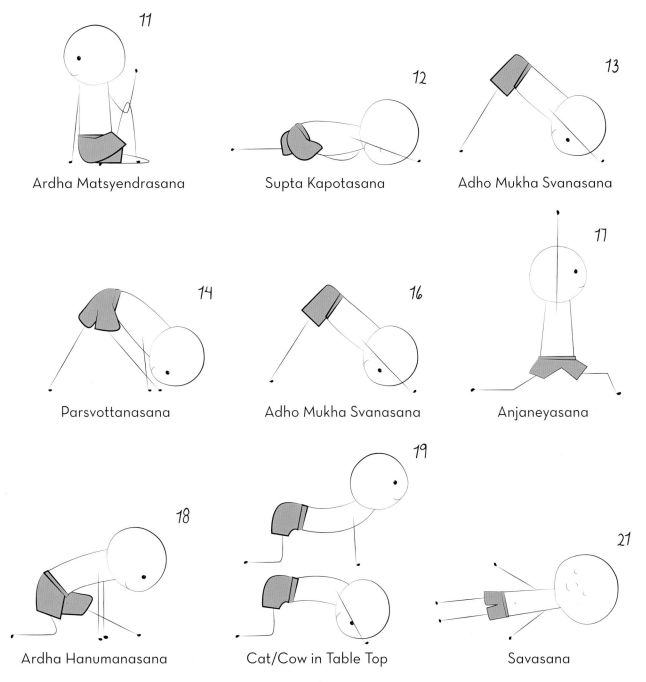

11 Ardha Matsyendrasana

12 Supta Kapotasana

13 Adho Mukha Svanasana

14 Parsvottanasana

16 Adho Mukha Svanasana

17 Anjaneyasana

18 Ardha Hanumanasana

19 Cat/Cow in Table Top

21 Savasana

To Your Health!

Yoga for Physical Well-Being

Yoga for Upper Back, Neck, and Shoulders

We all hold tension in different parts of our bodies. Some yogis grit their teeth as they sleep and end up with jaw pain, while others don't even realize their hands are clenched into fists as they wait in line at the grocery store. I hold every ounce of stress in my upper back, neck, and shoulders. There's a good reason this part of the body is sometimes called the Iron Cross. Consider this sequence your cure for the Iron Cross. Be patient with your muscles as they become less steel-like and more human, and breathe deeply into your entire rib cage.

1. *Balasana* (Child's Pose)
2. Table Top
3. Cat/Cow spine in Table Top
4. *Adho Mukha Svanasana* (Downward Facing Dog Pose)
5. *Uttanasana* (Standing Forward Fold). Note: Take your hands to opposite elbows and let your torso sway.
6. *Tadasana* (Mountain Pose)
7. *Natarajasana* (Dancer's Pose)
8. *Virabhadrasana III* (Warrior III)
9. *Alanasana* (High Lunge Pose)
10. *Parivrtta Alanasana* (Twisted High Lunge Pose)
11. *Alanasana*

Turn to page 150 to complete sequence.

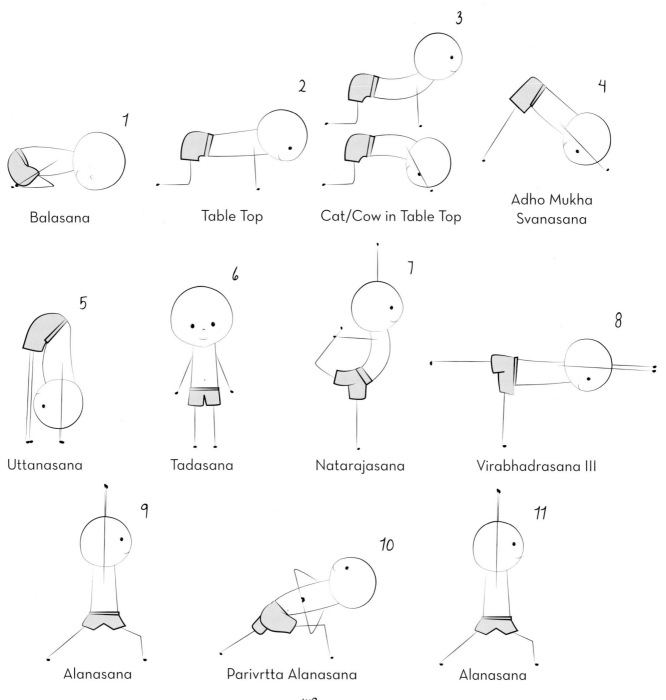

1 Balasana

2 Table Top

3 Cat/Cow in Table Top

4 Adho Mukha Svanasana

5 Uttanasana

6 Tadasana

7 Natarajasana

8 Virabhadrasana III

9 Alanasana

10 Parivrtta Alanasana

11 Alanasana

12. *Virabhadrasana II* (Warrior II Pose)

13. *Baddha Virabhadrasana* (Humble Warrior Pose)

14. *Prasarita Padottanasana* (Wide-Legged Forward Bend)

15. Repeat steps 6–14 on other side

16. *Tadasana*

17. *Bhujangasana* (Cobra Pose). Repeat a second time.

18. *Dhanurasana* (Bow Pose)

19. *Balasana*

20. *Paschimottanasana* (Seated Forward Fold)

21. *Supta Matsyendrasana* (Reclined Twist Pose). Repeat other side.

22. *Savasana* (Corpse Pose)

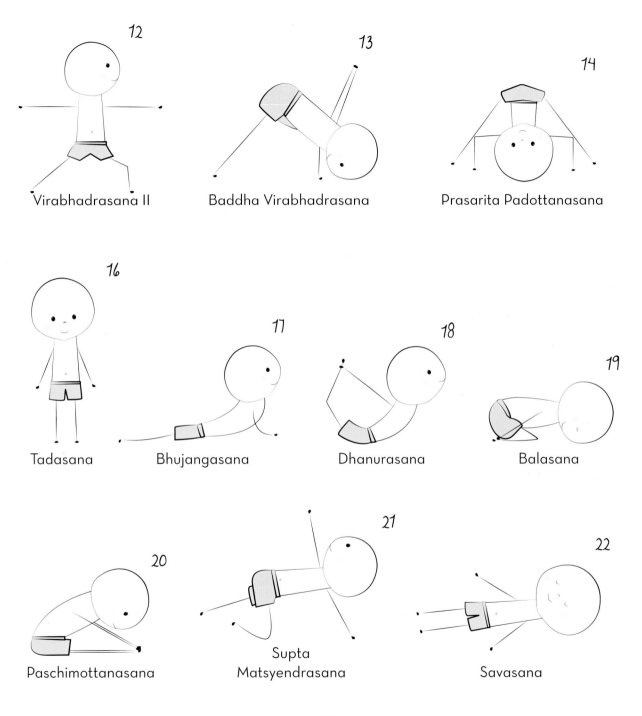

12 Virabhadrasana II

13 Baddha Virabhadrasana

14 Prasarita Padottanasana

16 Tadasana

17 Bhujangasana

18 Dhanurasana

19 Balasana

20 Paschimottanasana

21 Supta Matsyendrasana

22 Savasana

Yoga for Achy Lower Back and Hips

I teach one of my classes like a call-in radio show. At the beginning of class, I go around the room and ask everyone what they want to work on, whether it be a particular pose or a part of the body. In theory, it looks like I'm planning the class on the fly. In reality, someone always ends up mentioning the hips and lower back, so I build it into the class plan before I even walk into the studio. If this is an ache you experience on a regular basis, rest knowing you are not alone. After this sequence, your muscles can finally get a rest, too.

1. *Tadasana* (Mountain Pose)

2. *Uttanasana* (Standing Forward Fold). Note: Be careful to bend at the hips and not at the stomach.

3. *Trikonasana* (Triangle Pose)

4. *Utthita Parsvakonasana* (Extended Side Angle Pose)

5. *Virabhadrasana II* (Warrior II)

6. Repeat steps 3-5 on other side

7. *Supta Kapotasana* (Reclined Pigeon Pose). Repeat on other side. Note: Use bolsters, if needed, to keep hips aligned.

8. *Bhujangasana* (Cobra Pose)

Turn to page 154 to complete sequence.

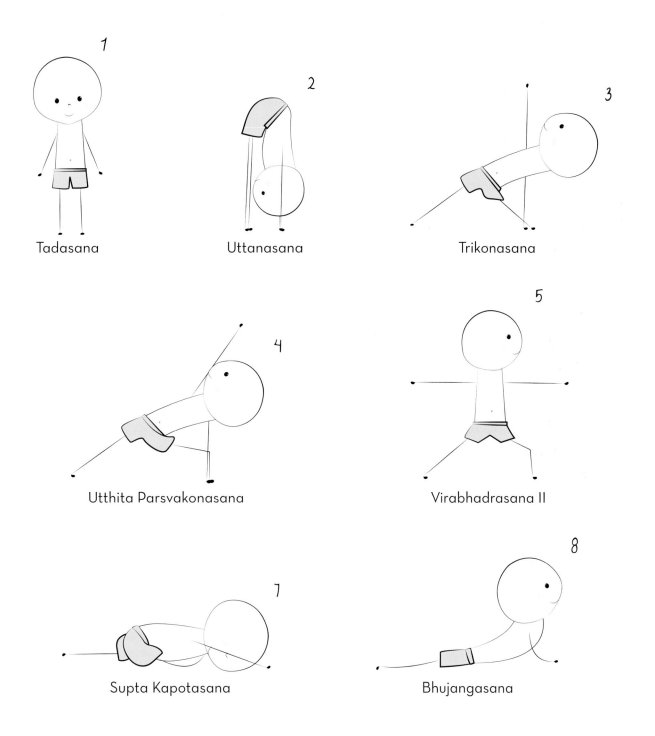

1
Tadasana

2
Uttanasana

3
Trikonasana

4
Utthita Parsvakonasana

5
Virabhadrasana II

7
Supta Kapotasana

8
Bhujangasana

9. *SALABHASANA* (Locust Pose)

10. *DHANURASANA* (Bow Pose)

11. *BALASANA* (Child's Pose)

12. *VAJRASANA* (Diamond Pose)

13. *GOMUKHASANA* (Cow Face Pose). Repeat on other side.

14. *JANU SIRSASANA* (Head to Knee Pose). Repeat on other side.

15. *ANANDA BALASANA* (Happy Baby Pose)

16. *SAVASANA* (Corpse Pose)

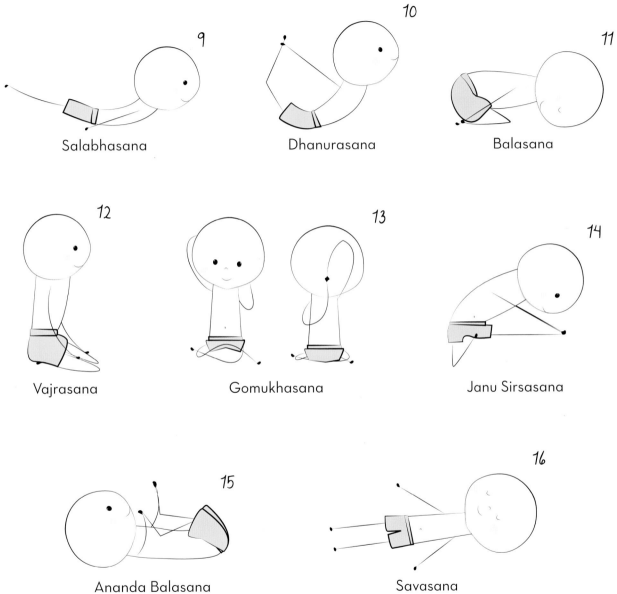

9 Salabhasana

10 Dhanurasana

11 Balasana

12 Vajrasana

13 Gomukhasana

14 Janu Sirsasana

15 Ananda Balasana

16 Savasana

Yoga to Relieve Sinus Pressure

Let's say you forgot to do your Immunity Boosting Sequence from the first chapter. Unfortunately, you came down with a little bit of a cold, and now it feels like your sinuses are about to explode. Now what? Good thing yoga forgives all lapses in practice and has a cure for this, too. I know the impulse is going to be to keep your head upright, and we'll do that for the beginning of this sequence while we gently stimulate the movement of lymph. Then, a long inversion like Shoulderstand allows the pressure to build and build and build . . . before totally and deliciously releasing. Ah, feels nice to breathe again!

1. *TADASANA* (Mountain Pose)
2. *VIRABHADRASANA I* (Warrior I Pose). Repeat with other leg.
3. *VIRABHADRASANA II* (Warrior II Pose)
4. *TRIKONASANA* (Triangle Pose)
5. Repeat steps 3 and 4 on other side
6. *TADASANA*
7. *PASCHIMOTTANASANA* (Seated Forward Fold)
8. *SARVANGASANA* (Shoulderstand Pose). Hold for 3-5 minutes. Note: Use bolsters and make into supported shoulderstand if desired.
9. *HALASANA* (Plow Pose). Hold for 1-2 minutes. Note: Again, use props as desired.
10. *SUPTA MATSYENDRASANA* (Reclined Twist Pose). Repeat other side.
11. *SAVASANA* (Corpse Pose)

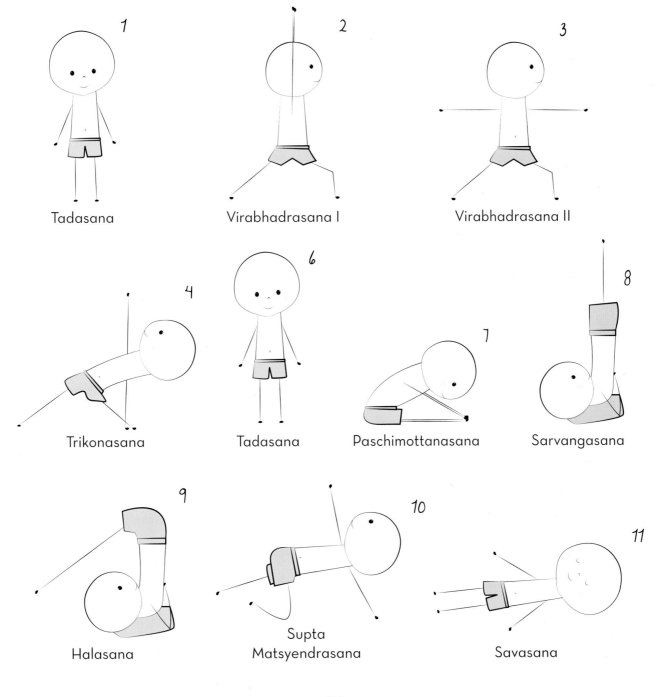

1 Tadasana

2 Virabhadrasana I

3 Virabhadrasana II

4 Trikonasana

6 Tadasana

7 Paschimottanasana

8 Sarvangasana

9 Halasana

10 Supta Matsyendrasana

11 Savasana

Yoga for Sensitive Wrists

I get something on my right wrist called a ganglion cyst, but my doctor calls it a Bible bump. Curious as to why? One way to get rid of it is to hit the cyst with the heaviest book in your home, like the Bible. Needless to say, it hurts so much you see stars. In my experience, I find yoga to be a gentler solution. When I practice with care and attention to my wrists, I find better results than I could with any violent action with a book. If you have any other kind of wrist trouble (repetitive stress, carpal tunnel syndrome, arthritis—just to name a few), you might find that yoga is just the cure you need.

1. *BALASANA* (Child's Pose)
2. Table Top on forearms. Note: Focus on pressing into the thumb and pointer finger to strengthen and align the wrist muscles without straining them.
3. Cat/Cow spine in Table Top on forearms
4. Dolphin Pose
5. *UTTANASANA* (Standing Forward Fold)
6. *URDHVA HASTASANA* (Upward Hands Pose)
7. *NATARAJASANA* (Dancer's Pose). Repeat on other side.
8. *VIRABHARASANA III* (Warrior III Pose). Repeat on other side.
9. *GARUNDASANA* (Eagle Pose). Repeat on other side.

TURN TO PAGE 160 TO COMPLETE SEQUENCE.

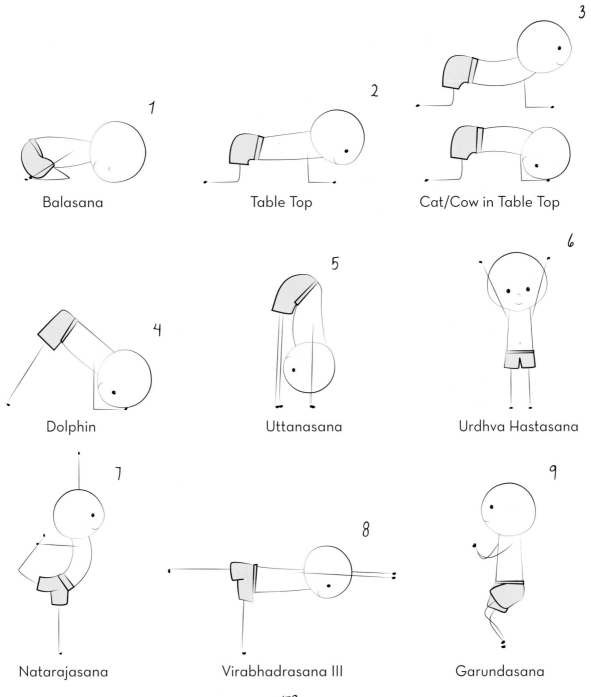

1 Balasana

2 Table Top

3 Cat/Cow in Table Top

4 Dolphin

5 Uttanasana

6 Urdhva Hastasana

7 Natarajasana

8 Virabhadrasana III

9 Garundasana

10. *YOGA MUDRASANA* (Standing fold with hands interlaced behind back)

11. *UTKATASANA* (Chair Pose)

12. *PARIVRTTA UTKATASANA* (Revolved Chair Pose). Repeat on other side.

13. *UTTANASANA* (Standing Forward Fold)

14. *MALASANA* (Seated Squat Pose)

15. *GOMUKHASANA* (Cow Face Pose). Repeat on other side.

16. *ARDHA MATSYENDRASANA* (Half Seated Twist Pose). Repeat on other side.

17. *HALASANA* (Plow Pose)

18. *SAVASANA* (Corpse Pose)

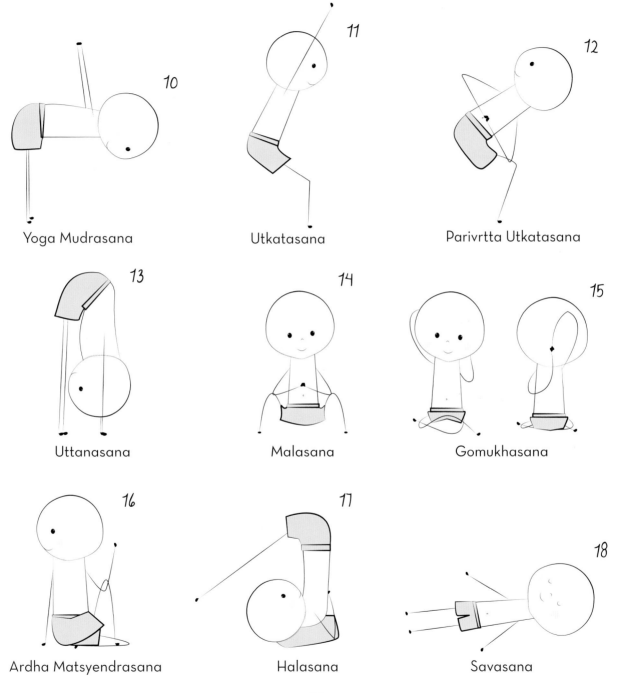

10 Yoga Mudrasana

11 Utkatasana

12 Parivrtta Utkatasana

13 Uttanasana

14 Malasana

15 Gomukhasana

16 Ardha Matsyendrasana

17 Halasana

18 Savasana

Yoga for Stomachaches

Ever eat some sketchy street food while adventure traveling and quickly regret it? I've been there, done that, and frankly recommend that you lie down and hydrate yourself well. This is a sequence for general indigestion (gas, nausea, bloating, etc.) on a lesser scale. If something isn't working for what's ailing you, however, you'll know pretty fast. Don't push yourself through it.

1. *SUKHASANA* (Easy Pose)
2. *NADI SHODANA PRANAYAMA* (Alternate Nostril Breathing). Continue for 10 minutes.
3. *BALASANA* (Child's Pose). Hold for 5-10 breaths.
4. *BADDHA KONASANA* (Bound Angle Pose)
5. *JANU SIRSASANA* (Head to Knee Pose). Repeat on other side.
6. *SUPTA PAVANA MUKTASANA* (Reclined Wind Relieving Pose). Repeat on other side.
7. *SUPTA MATSYENDRASANA* (Reclined Twist Pose). Repeat on other side.
8. *APANASANA* (Knees to Chest on Back)
9. *SAVASANA* (Corpse Pose)

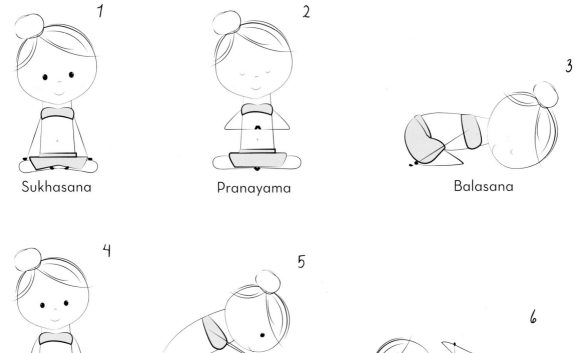

1
Sukhasana

2
Pranayama

3
Balasana

4
Baddha Konasana

5
Janu Sirsasana

6
Supta Pavana Muktasana

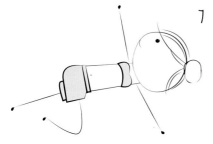

7
Supta Matsyendrasana

8
Apanasana

9
Savasana

Yoga for Hangovers

My guess is that if you're reading this paragraph, the last thing you want to do is pull out your yoga mat. Maybe you want to curl in a ball, draw the shades, and take the day off. Sorry, but the quickest way out of this suffering is to drag yourself out of bed and onto the mat. Think about it: If you were doing yoga all last night instead of what you were actually doing, you wouldn't be in this mess, would you? Yoga will move the detoxification process along and help sweat out some of your misery.

1. *Vajrasana* (Diamond Pose)
2. *Ardha Matsyendrasana* (Half Seated Twist Pose). Repeat other direction.
3. *Tadasana* (Mountain Pose)
4. *Pavana Muktasana* (Standing Wind Relieving Pose). Repeat on other side.
5. *Uttanasana* (Standing Forward Fold)
6. *Malasana* (Seated Squat Pose)
7. *Paschimottanasana* (Seated Forward Fold)
8. *Supta Pavana Muktasana* (Reclined Wind Relieving Pose). Repeat on other side.

Turn to page 166 to complete sequence.

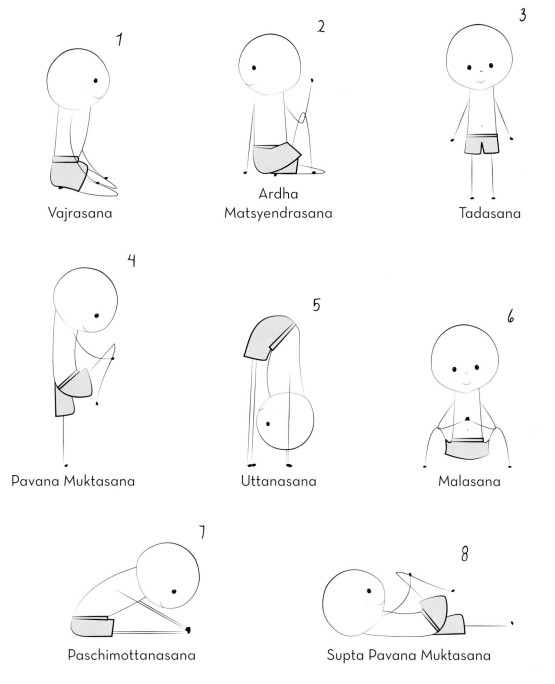

1 Vajrasana

2 Ardha Matsyendrasana

3 Tadasana

4 Pavana Muktasana

5 Uttanasana

6 Malasana

7 Paschimottanasana

8 Supta Pavana Muktasana

165

9. *Apanasana* (Knees to Chest on Back)

10. *Supta Matsyendrasana* (Reclined Twist Pose). Repeat on other side.

11. *Sarvangasana* (Shoulderstand Pose)

12. *Halasana* (Plow Pose)

13. *Matsyasana* (Fish Pose)

14. *Sirsasana* (Headstand Pose)

15. *Balasana* (Child's Pose)

16. *Savasana* (Corpse Pose)

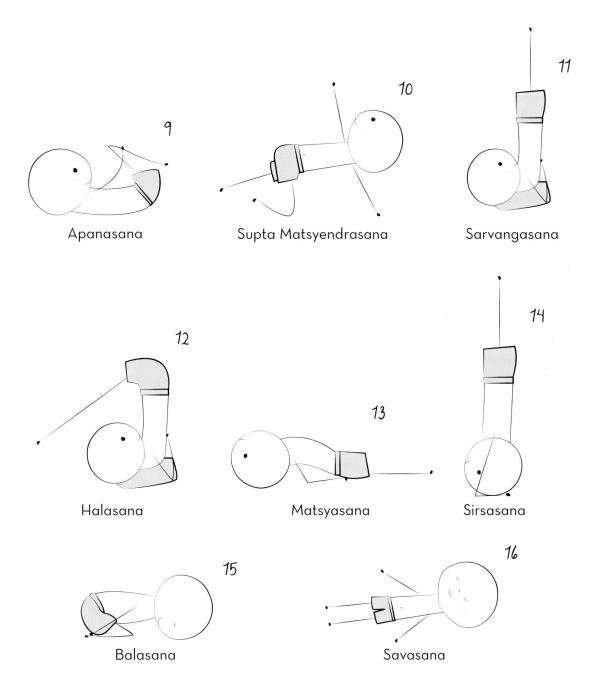

9

Apanasana

10

Supta Matsyendrasana

11

Sarvangasana

12

Halasana

13

Matsyasana

14

Sirsasana

15

Balasana

16

Savasana

This Is Your Brain on Yoga

Yoga for Mental Health

Yoga for Heartbreak

When something emotionally devastating happens, whether it be the dissolution of a relationship or a loved one's passing, it can feel like our hearts are literally falling apart, right there in our chests. As someone who has experienced her fair share of heartbreak, I adopted a new strategy. Instead of seeing my heart as something broken (like some piece of machinery), I try to see my heart broken open to let in new understanding, light, and truth. Remember: our hearts feel broken because we loved fully, which is never a bad thing. Here is a practice to help encourage you to keep that heart broken open and resist the temptation to put up barriers. You'll be glad you did.

1. *SUKHASANA* (Easy Pose). Note: Take one hand to heart and one hand to belly. Breathe into both of your hands.
2. *ANAHATASANA* (Extended Puppy Dog Pose)
3. Table Top
4. *VYAGHRASANA* (Tiger Pose). Repeat on other side.
5. *BALASANA* (Child's Pose)
6. *ADHO MUKHA SVANASANA* (Downward Facing Dog Pose)
7. *UTTANASANA* (Standing Forward Fold)
8. *TADASANA* (Mountain Pose)
9. *VIRABHADRASANA I* (Warrior I Pose)

TURN TO PAGE 172 TO COMPLETE SEQUENCE.

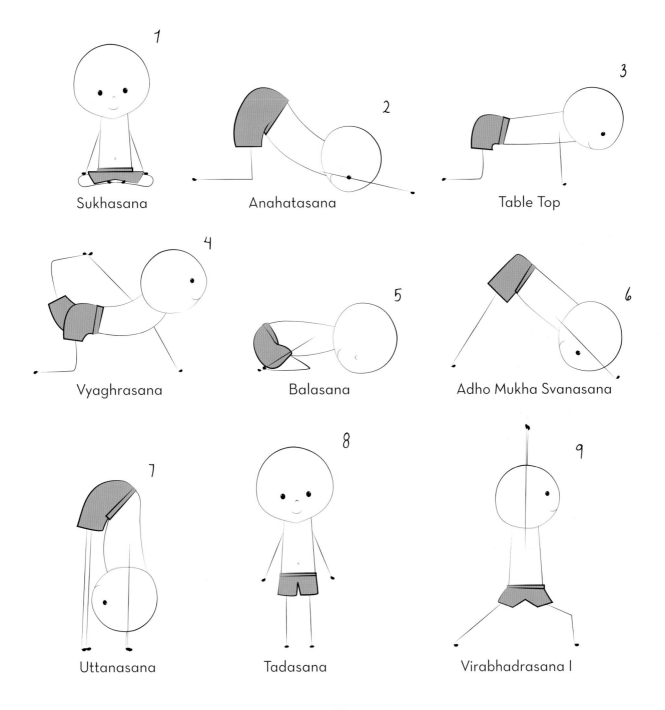

1 Sukhasana

2 Anahatasana

3 Table Top

4 Vyaghrasana

5 Balasana

6 Adho Mukha Svanasana

7 Uttanasana

8 Tadasana

9 Virabhadrasana I

10. *Baddha Virabhadrasana* (Humble Warrior Pose)

11. *Parsvottanasana* (Intense Stretch Pose)

12. *Trikonasana* (Triangle Pose)

13. Repeat steps 9–12 with other leg

14. *Vrksasana* (Tree Pose). Repeat on other side.

15. *Setu Bandhasana* (Bridge Pose). Note: Either repeat *Setu Bandhasana* or come into *Urdhva Dhanurasana* (Wheel Pose) for a second heart opener.

16. *Paschimottanasana* (Seated Forward Fold)

17. *Janu Sirsasana* (Head to Knee Pose). Repeat on other side.

18. *Ardha Matsyendrasana* (Half Seated Twist Pose). Repeat on other side.

19. *Savasana* (Corpse Pose)

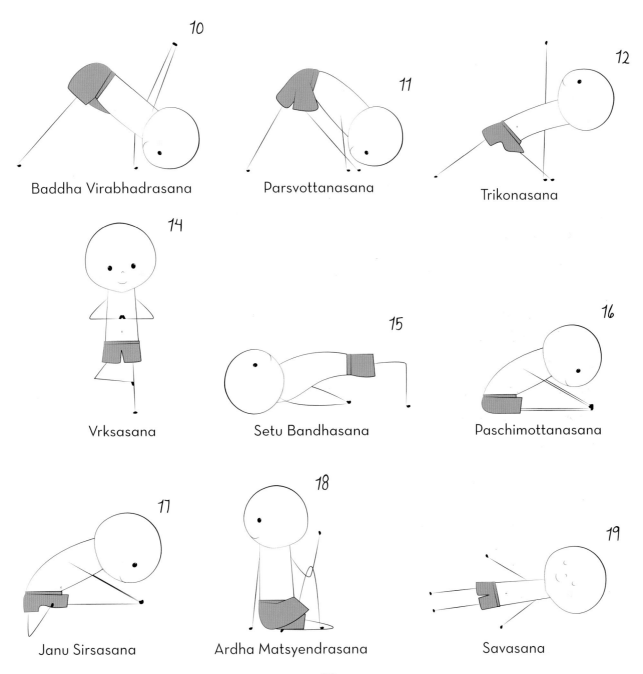

Baddha Virabhadrasana

Parsvottanasana

Trikonasana

Vrksasana

Setu Bandhasana

Paschimottanasana

Janu Sirsasana

Ardha Matsyendrasana

Savasana

Yoga for Balance

You know the best thing about yoga poses that strengthen your physical balance? They bring mental balance, too. Allowing yourself to be still and focused drops your blood pressure, slows your breathing, and reduces the release of stress hormones. Remember to breathe evenly and easily and you'll find that not only is your Tree Pose relaxed but so is your mind.

1. *SUKHASANA* (Easy Pose)
2. *DIRGHA PRANAYAMA* (Three Part Yogic Breath)
3. *JANU SIRSASANA* (Head to Knee Pose). Repeat on both sides.
4. *TADASANA* (Mountain Pose)
5. *VRKASANA* (Tree Pose). Repeat on other side.
6. *TADASANA*
7. *PAVANA MUKTASANA* (Standing Wind Relieving Pose). Repeat on other side.

TURN TO PAGE 176 TO COMPLETE SEQUENCE.

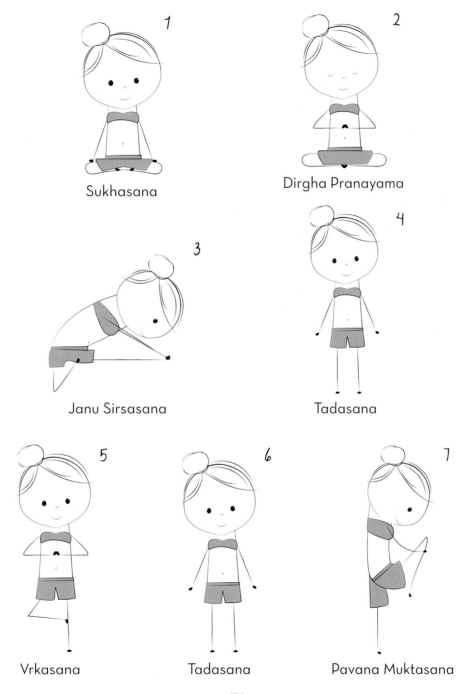

1 Sukhasana

2 Dirgha Pranayama

3 Janu Sirsasana

4 Tadasana

5 Vrkasana

6 Tadasana

7 Pavana Muktasana

8. *Tadasana*

9. *Virabhadrasana I* (Warrior I Pose)

10. *Virabhadrasana III* (Warrior III Pose)

11. Repeat steps 9 and 10 on other side

12. Plank Pose

13. *Vasisthasana* (Side Plank Pose). Repeat on other side.

14. *Bhujangasana* (Cobra Pose). Repeat.

15. *Savasana* (Corpse Pose)

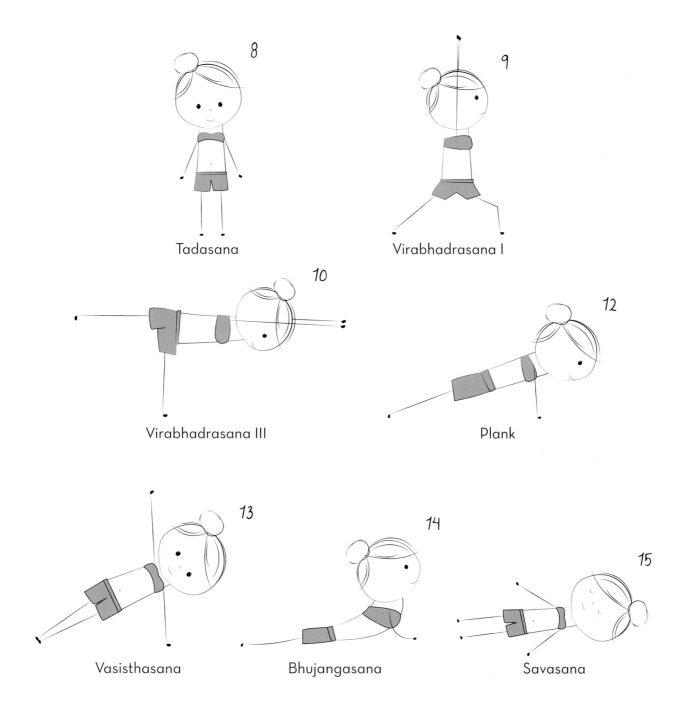

8 Tadasana

9 Virabhadrasana I

10 Virabhadrasana III

12 Plank

13 Vasisthasana

14 Bhujangasana

15 Savasana

Yoga for Gratitude

Every year around Thanksgiving I teach a class based on the following mantra (attributed to the Zen master Sono): "Thank you for everything. I have no complaint(s) whatsoever." I have found that when things are amazing, it feels amazing to affirm my gratitude. I have also found that when things are less than amazing, it feels grounding and peaceful to say the same mantra. We cannot only be grateful when everything is peaches and cream. Anyway, who are we to say what is a blessing and what is a curse? I'm sure we all have situations in our past that we lamented at the time, but can now see that they unfolded exactly as they should have. And vice versa.

As you practice this sequence, I invite you to meditate on everything that you are grateful for at this moment. Let every breath in fill you with gratitude and every breath out be a reminder that you can take nothing for granted. If you have a mantra, you can say that in your mind. As for me, I'm sticking with the old standard: THANK YOU FOR EVERYTHING. I HAVE NO COMPLAINTS WHATSOEVER.

1. *VAJRASANA* (Diamond Pose)
2. *GOMUKHASANA* (Cow Face Pose). Repeat on other side.
3. *VIRASANA* (Heroes Pose)
4. *SUPTA VIRASANA* (Reclined Heroes Pose). Note: Use lots of props under body, as needed.
5. Cat/Cow spine in Table Top
6. *ARDHA MATSYENDRASANA* (Half Seated Twist Pose). Repeat on other side.
7. *ANAHATASANA* (Extended Puppy Dog Pose)
8. *ADHO MUKHA SVANASANA* (Downward Facing Dog Pose)
9. *SUPTA KAPOTASANA* (Reclined Pigeon Pose)
10. Repeat steps 7-9 on other side

TURN TO PAGE 180 TO CONTINUE SEQUENCE.

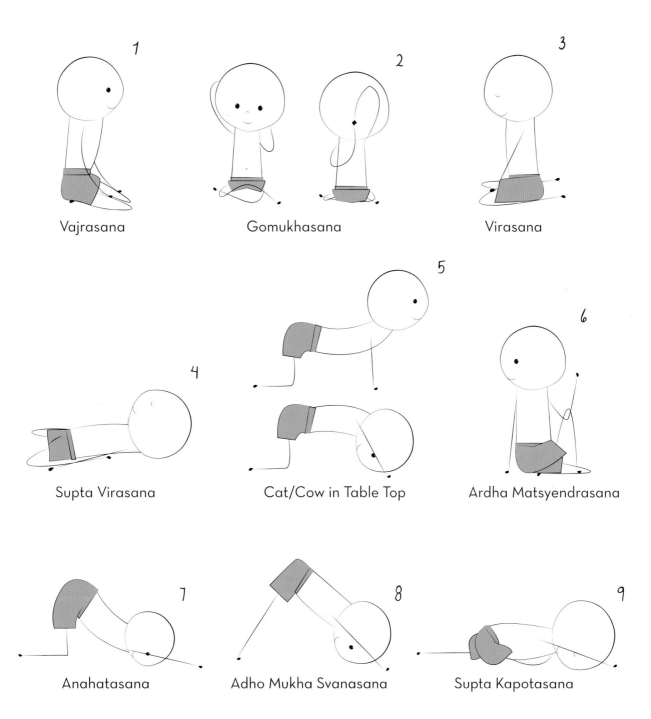

1 Vajrasana

2 Gomukhasana

3 Virasana

4 Supta Virasana

5 Cat/Cow in Table Top

6 Ardha Matsyendrasana

7 Anahatasana

8 Adho Mukha Svanasana

9 Supta Kapotasana

11. *TADASANA* (Mountain Pose)

12. *UTTANASANA* (Standing Forward Fold)

13. *URDHVA HASTASANA* (Upward Hands Pose). Note: Reach one hand higher and then the other, stretching the sides of your body.

14. *PARSVOTTANASANA* (Intense Side Stretch Pose). Repeat on other side.

15. *URDHVA HASTASANA*

16. *TADASANA*

TURN TO PAGE 182 TO COMPLETE SEQUENCE.

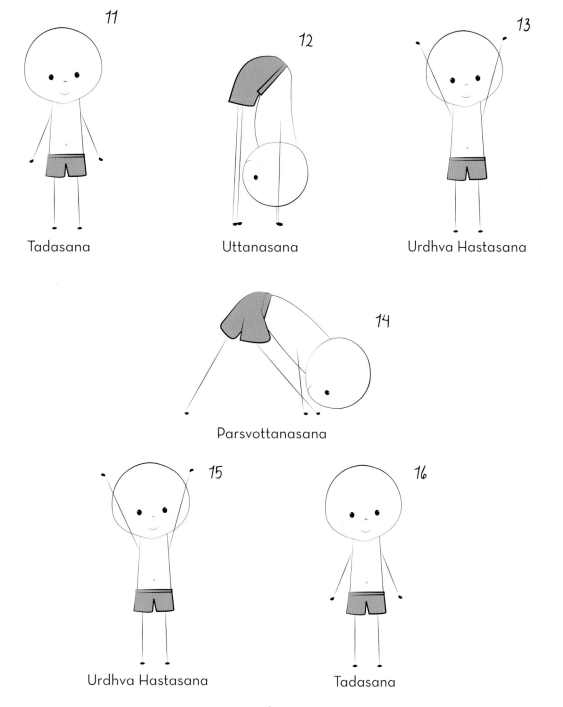

11 Tadasana

12 Uttanasana

13 Urdhva Hastasana

14 Parsvottanasana

15 Urdhva Hastasana

16 Tadasana

17. *Natarajasana* (Dancer's Pose). Repeat on other side.

18. *Prasarita Padottanasana* (Wide-Legged Forward Bend). Note: Interlock fingers behind back to get a back and shoulder stretch as well.

19. *Janu Sirsasana* (Head to Knee Pose)

20. *Upavistha Konasana* (Seated Wide Angle Pose)

21. Repeat steps 19 and 20 on other side

22. *Supta Matsyendrasana* (Reclined Twist Pose). Repeat on other side.

23. *Savasana* (Corpse Pose)

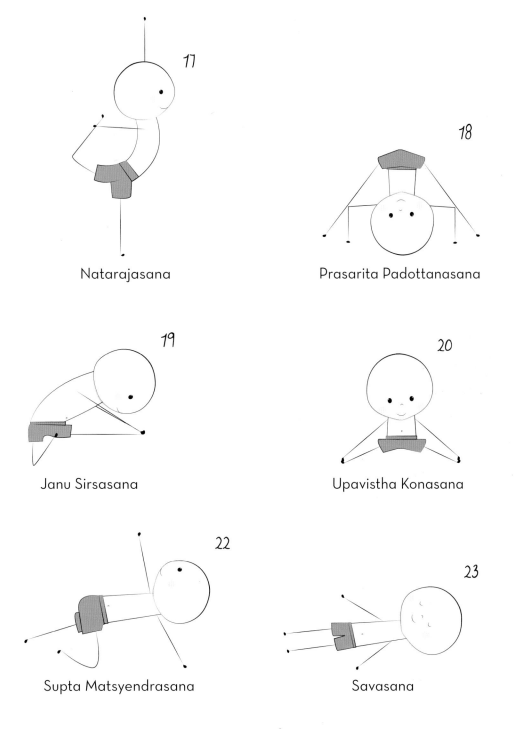

17 Natarajasana

18 Prasarita Padottanasana

19 Janu Sirsasana

20 Upavistha Konasana

22 Supta Matsyendrasana

23 Savasana

Yoga to Create More Space, Mentally and Physically

Close your eyes. In your mind, take a moment and envision five pairs of shoes you own. See the colors, shapes, and their current location. Think about where you bought them. Think about how much they cost and the story behind acquiring them.

You may be thinking, *SHOES*? But here's the point: if you can close your eyes and imagine five pairs of shoes (personally, I can see a whole lot more than five, just from where I'm sitting right now), that means that in addition to taking up space in your closet, the shoes are also *TAKING UP SPACE IN YOUR CONSCIOUSNESS*. This shoe experiment can be repeated on coats, bags, silverware, coffee mugs, etc. All of this stuff is just lying in our minds, gathering dust.

Take the time before you practice yoga to create a clean, comfortable space in which to practice. Remove physical distractions, shut off your phone, and forget about all those shoes. If you clear your physical space before you practice, you'll be surprised by how much easier it is to make more space in your mind.

1. *SIMHASANA PRANAYAMA* (Lion's Breath)
2. Knee-down *TADASANA* (Mountain Pose)
3. *PARIGHASANA* (Gate Pose). Note: Swing the non-planted hand in circles about you.
4. Cat/Cow spine in Table Top
5. Repeat steps 2–4 on other side
6. *ADHO MUKHA SVANASANA* (Downward Facing Dog Pose) Note: Lift one leg into Three-legged Dog, drawing circles with non-planted knee. Repeat other side.
7. *UTTANASANA* (Standing Forward Fold)

TURN TO PAGE 186 TO CONTINUE SEQUENCE.

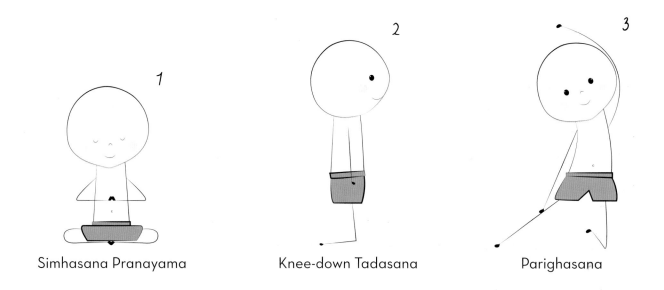

1	*2*	*3*
Simhasana Pranayama	Knee-down Tadasana	Parighasana

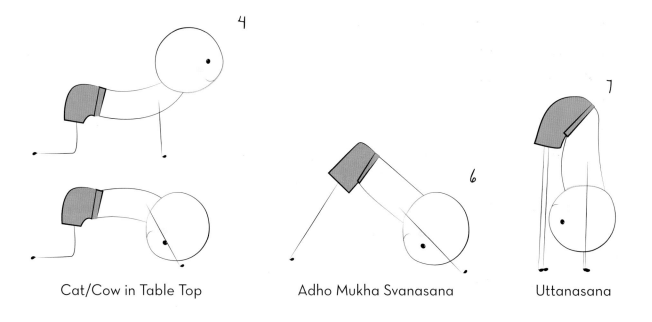

4	*6*	*7*
Cat/Cow in Table Top	Adho Mukha Svanasana	Uttanasana

8. *Urdhva Hastasana* (Upward Hands Pose). Hold for 10 cycles of breaths.

9. *Virabhadrasana III* (Warrior III Pose)

10. *Virabhadrasana I* (Warrior I Pose)

11. *Virabhadrasana II* (Warrior II Pose)

12. Repeat steps 6-11

13. *Prasarita Padottanasana* (Wide-Legged Forward Bend)

14. *Deviasana* (Goddess Pose or Horse Stance). Hold for 10 cycles of breaths.

15. *Urdhva Hastasana*

Turn to page 188 to complete sequence.

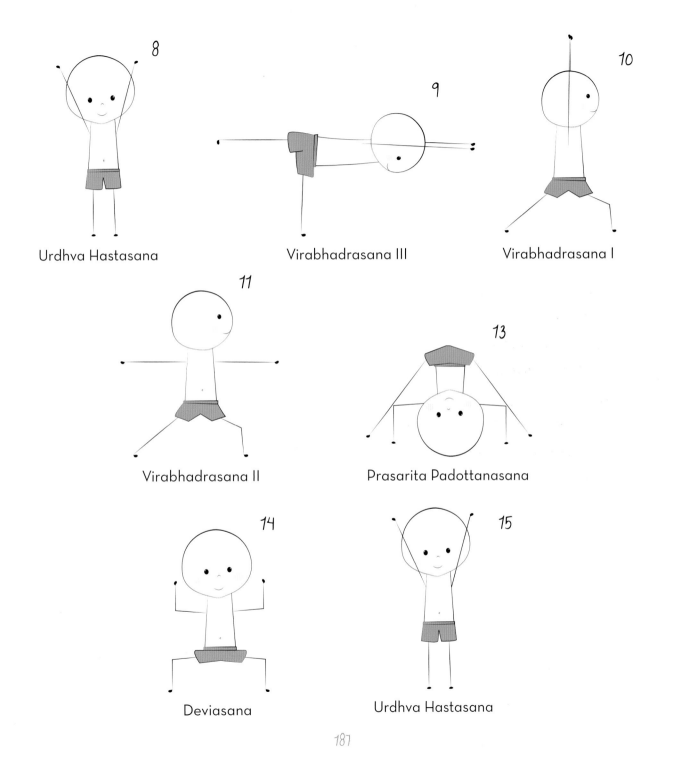

8 Urdhva Hastasana

9 Virabhadrasana III

10 Virabhadrasana I

11 Virabhadrasana II

13 Prasarita Padottanasana

14 Deviasana

15 Urdhva Hastasana

16. *BALASANA* (Child's Pose)

17. *DHANURASANA* (Bow Pose)

18. *BALASANA*

19. *SARVANGASANA* (Shoulderstand Pose)

20. *HALASANA* (Plow Pose)

21. *SUPTA MATSYENDRASANA* (Reclined Twist Pose). Repeat other side.

22. *SAVASANA* (Corpse Pose)

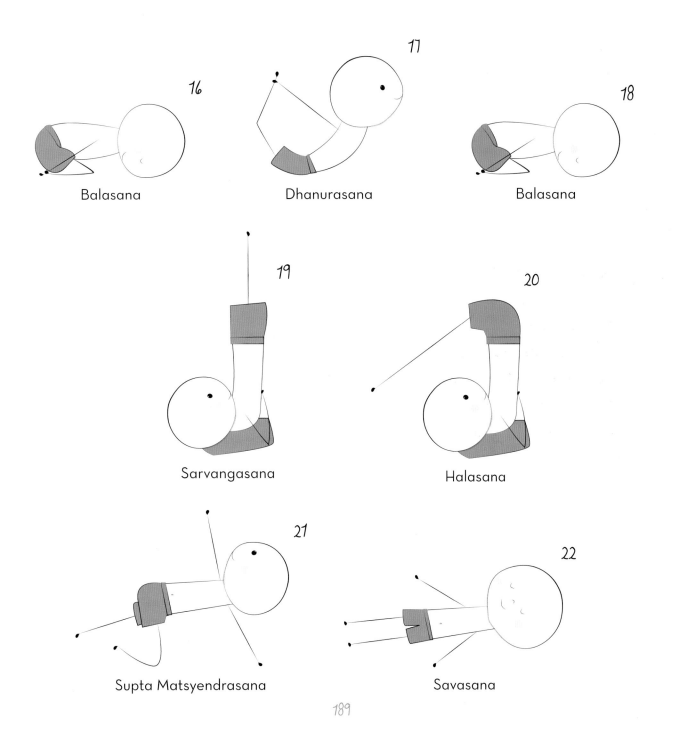

16

Balasana

17

Dhanurasana

18

Balasana

19

Sarvangasana

20

Halasana

21

Supta Matsyendrasana

22

Savasana

Yoga for Sad Days

"Someone I loved once gave me a box full of darkness. It took me years to understand that this, too, was a gift."— Mary Oliver

We all have sad days. Sometimes we know why, sometimes we don't. Often, on these sad days, our instincts aren't at their best. While you might want to hide from the world with a sappy movie and a hankie, a yoga practice can help reduce the release of cortisol (a stress hormone) and activate the sympathetic nervous system—which can really help brighten your mood. Yoga can help these sad days be a gift to a greater understanding of your body and a path to more patience with your mind.

1. *Supta Baddha Konasana* (Reclined Bound Angle Pose). Note: Use props under the torso, head, and neck as needed.
2. *Supta Matsyendrasana* (Reclined Twist Pose). Repeat on other side.
3. *Setu Bandhasana* (Bridge Pose)
4. *Balasana* (Child's Pose)
5. *Adho Mukha Svanasana* (Downward Facing Dog Pose)
6. *Prasarita Padottanasana* (Wide-Legged Forward Bend)
7. *Urdhva Hastasana* (Upward Hands Pose)
8. *Tadasana* (Mountain Pose)
9. *Vrksasana* (Tree Pose). Repeat on other side.

Turn to page 192 to complete sequence.

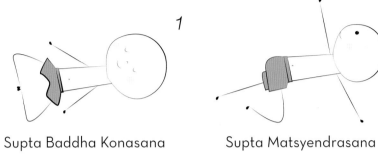

1

Supta Baddha Konasana

2

Supta Matsyendrasana

3

Setu Bandhasana

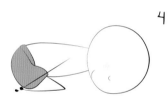

4

Balasana

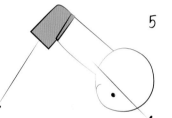

5

Adho Mukha Svanasana

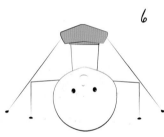

6

Prasarita Padottanasana

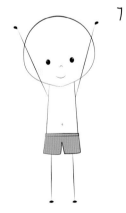

7

Urdhva Hastasana

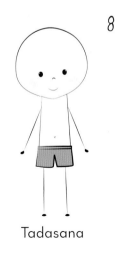

8

Tadasana

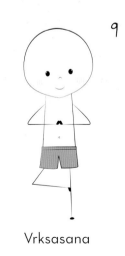

9

Vrksasana

10. *VIRABHADRASANA III* (Warrior III Pose). Repeat on other side.

11. *ARDHA CHANDRASANA* (Balancing Half Moon Pose). Repeat on other side. Note: Practice this pose with your back against the wall if you feel off balance physically.

12. *PASCHIMOTTANASANA* (Seated Forward Fold)

13. *SARVANGASANA* (Shoulderstand Pose)

14. *HALASANA* (Plow Pose)

15. *MATSYASANA* (Fish Pose)

16. *SIRSASANA* (Headstand Pose)

17. *SAVASANA* (Corpse Pose)

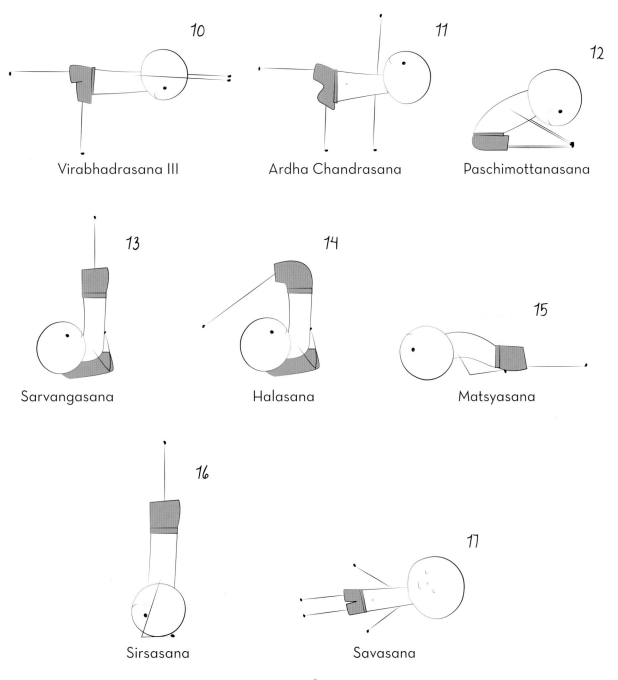

10 Virabhadrasana III

11 Ardha Chandrasana

12 Paschimottanasana

13 Sarvangasana

14 Halasana

15 Matsyasana

16 Sirsasana

17 Savasana

193

Yoga for Anger Management

Years ago, I was housesitting for my parents while my younger brother (who couldn't housesit a birdhouse) was living at home. We got into an argument and I left the house. When I returned home, he had taken out every single pot and pan, placed them on the kitchen counters . . . and covered them in ketchup. My first plan of action was to take all the pans and tuck them neatly into his bed (hello, *GODFATHER*). I had to teach a yoga class first, however, and planned to enact revenge when I got home.

Maybe you can predict where this story is going. Just by teaching a yoga class, and becoming more aware of my uneven breathing, agitated mind, and racing pulse, I knew that revenge was not the best solution. When I got home, I cleaned all the pots and pans and was pleasantly surprised to notice that ketchup acts as a deep cleaner for copper and brass cookware. In the end, my mind (and the pots) was shinier than ever. By focusing on remedying some of the side effects of being really mad, the anger itself will dissolve faster than ketchup.

1. Seated Meditation. Note: Focus on evening out the breath to equal inhale and exhale lengths.
2. *NADI SHODANA PRANAYAMA* (Alternate Nostril Breathing). Practice for 5-15 minutes.
3. *SIMHASANA PRANAYAMA* (Lion's Breath)
4. Cat/Cow spine in Table Top, moving with the breath
5. *BHUJANGASANA* (Cobra Pose)
6. *SALABHASANA* (Locust Pose)
7. *BALASANA* (Child's Pose). Hold for 1-3 minutes.
8. *PASCHIMOTTANASANA* (Seated Forward Fold)
9. *JANU SIRSASANA* (Head to Knee Pose). Repeat other side.
10. *HALASANA* (Plow Pose)
11. *VIPARITA KARANI* (Legs up the Wall Pose). Hold for 5-15 minutes.
12. *SAVASANA* (Corpse Pose)

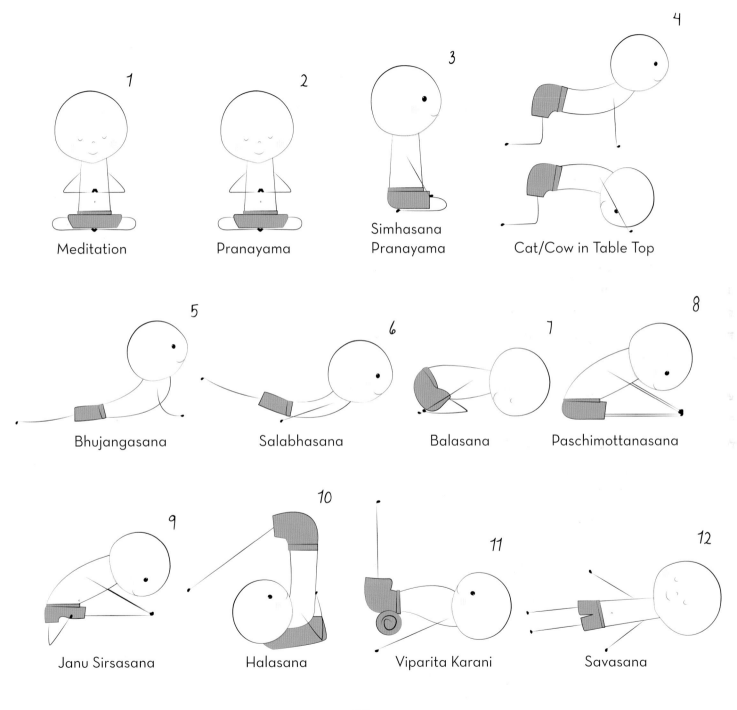

1 Meditation

2 Pranayama

3 Simhasana Pranayama

4 Cat/Cow in Table Top

5 Bhujangasana

6 Salabhasana

7 Balasana

8 Paschimottanasana

9 Janu Sirsasana

10 Halasana

11 Viparita Karani

12 Savasana

Acknowledgments

My mom and I both admit to always reading the acknowledgments page of books. Neither of us are entirely sure why. For all of you voracious acknowledgment readers out there (I imagine we are a club with few members), I acknowledge you, and will try to make this as entertaining as possible.

To the dynamic and brilliant sister team of Kerri and Nicole Frail. I would have considered myself blessed with one Frail, and I found myself with two. This book exists because of the both of you. I am equally grateful to my agent, Kathleen Rushall. You are patient, persistent, and so amazingly on top of everything.

In 2007, this book began as an idea at the Kripalu Center for Yoga and Health. My gratitude to Kripalu for SEVA, YTT, and Devarshi and Sudha. Since then, I've sought out the advice of many. F-stop Fitzgerald, Naomi Silverman, and Larry Bush were invaluable resources—people who actually knew what they were doing.

To my former and current employers: Emily Yachinich and Diane Fine of Cornell University, Tory Jenis at Blackbird Yoga, and Heather Healey at Mighty Yoga. I have amazing role models in professionalism, balance, and how to use a headset. In addition, my thanks to my co-teachers; I've learned so much from all of you.

And while this book wouldn't have been possible without the former people and communities, I wouldn't be who I am without the following incredible human beings (by timeline):

To my small, rowdy, and perfect family, especially Grandpa Manny, who saw a full century, but just missed the publishing of this book.

To Simon's Rock College of Bard (if you went there, you'd understand). To my soul friends Saro Hinson and Heather Fisch, my unofficial publicist Erica Webb, and her assistant Ashley Nelson.

To Sara Giffin, the adopted Silverman. To Madison's Friday night ladies' tea time.

To Colin Jermain, for your support on the front lines of this incredible process and for having a keen sense of aesthetics. To Chris Negronida, for being there in this project's infancy and believing that I could do it. Thank you both for sharing so much of this path with me; you have my love.

To Ithaca, New York. I tried to actually list out the people who have helped me in some way during this process, and I am so lucky to report that the list got out of hand pretty quickly. To amazing women: Ilana, Nicole, Emma, E-dub, Shoshi, Luisa, Tess, Jenna, Anaar, Dara, Kendra, Yardenne, Meg, and Megan. I love you, I love you, I love you.

Above all, my gratitude, love, and appreciation for my students, who are my teachers.

Thank you for everything; I have no complaints whatsoever.